# Challenging the Breast Cancer Legacy

# Challenging the Breast Cancer Legacy

## A PROGRAM OF EMOTIONAL SUPPORT
## AND MEDICAL CARE FOR WOMEN AT RISK

*Renee Royak-Schaler, Ph.D.*

AND

*Beryl Lieff Benderly*

HarperCollins*Publishers*

616.89
R 888c

HarperCollins books may be purchased for educational, business, or sales promotional use. For information, please call or write: Special Markets Department, HarperCollins Publishers, Inc., 10 East 53rd Street, New York, NY 10022.
Telephone: (212) 207-7528; Fax: (212) 207-7222.

FIRST EDITION

*Designed by Irving Perkins and Associates*

Royak-Schaler, Renee, 1946–
    Challenging the breast cancer legacy : a program of emotional
support and medical care for women at risk / Renee Royak-Schaler and
Beryl Lieff Benderly.—1st ed.
        p.  cm.
    Includes bibliographical references and index.
        ISBN 0-06-016625-8
        1. Breast—Cancer—Risk factors.   2. Breast—Cancer—Psychological
aspects.   3. Breast—Cancer—Prevention.   I. Benderly, Beryl Lieff.
II. Title.
    RC280.B8R69   1992
    616.99'449'0019—dc20                                                    91-50449

92  93  94  95  96  AC/HC  10  9  8  7  6  5  4  3  2  1

034897

## DEDICATED WITH LOVE

*to the memories of our grandmothers*

Rose Schanker Miller       Sarah Florin Jacobs
Celia Zimmerman Royak     Esther Pomerantz Lieff

*and to our mothers*

Sally Miller Royak       Pearl Jacobs Lieff

*sister*

Carla Royak Volturo

*daughters*

Magda Elise Schaler       Alicia Nadine Benderly

RRS     BLB

# Contents

*Contents*

## IV
### *A Program for Successful Living*

# Preface

❦

THIS BOOK grows out of the courage and generosity of thirty-two women. Each has at least one close relative (mother or sister) who has had breast cancer. And each agreed to speak candidly about the role that this disease plays in her own life—a difficult subject. We asked these women to explore their memories, reveal their feelings, and analyze the means they use to cope. Everyone who participated in the research projects from which this book grew did so in the spirit of helping her sisters everywhere. In that same spirit we offer the book.

In 1989, when this project began, very little research existed on women with strong family histories of breast cancer. Up to that time, the majority of psychosocial research on breast cancer had focused on the disease's impact on women patients and their families during the crisis of the illness. These studies emphasized the effects of treatments; the influence of social support from family, doctors, and other patients; and the coping styles that patients used.[1]

Between 1989 and 1991, a sample of eighty-five women coming to the Georgetown University Comprehensive Breast Center for routine checkups, evaluation, or treatment completed survey research questionnaires designed to explore their health practices, beliefs, and coping skills. A subset of this sample, thirty-two women, participated in a series of focus groups designed to elicit information and insights into both their experience with their mother's and/or sister's breast cancer and their reaction to their own elevated risk. The focus group format is a valuable research tool that encourages people to disclose their attitudes and behaviors related to a problem that concerns all the members. Focus groups afford a friendly, supportive environment in which participants perceive that all group members share some similar experiences, attitudes, and behaviors.[2]

Three different focus groups of about ten members each met for two sessions, lasting two hours each, conducted one week apart. Each of the thirty-two women participated in one set of these meetings. Guiding the discussions was a series of questions that elicited beliefs about breast cancer's significance, meaning, and causes and participants' emotional responses and coping skills during the relative's illness. A second set of questions then investigated what participants felt, thought, and did about their own high-risk status. This conversation also covered their coping skills and preventive health practices. The quotations in this book accurately reflect what was said in those sessions. The women's identities, however, have been disguised and some identifying details changed to protect their privacy.

Each participant felt a strong commitment to research that she believed could improve both the quality of life and the medical, social, and emotional services available to women at high risk. To this end, everyone conscientiously explored the meaning and significance of breast cancer in her life; the relationships between breast cancer and fear, hopelessness, and depression; and the strategies that she uses to cope with a disease that claims one woman in nine, is the number one killer of women between thirty and fifty, and is the number two cause of death of those over sixty.[3]

Participants were middle-class, college-educated Caucasian and African-American women with a mean age of forty-five. They showed a mixed record of following the health habits known to favor long life and good outcomes in breast cancer. Fully 96 percent complied with recommendations on clinical breast exams and 64 percent with recommendations on mammograms. But only 57 percent regularly practiced breast self-exam. Twenty-four percent chose low-fat diets, and 36 percent reduced their caffeine intake. Sixty percent eschewed alcohol and none smoked. Fifty-two percent exercised three or more times a week, the minimum necessary for fitness, and 33 percent successfully maintained a desirable weight for their height and body structure.

These data show that women practice the preventive health behaviors that are under their own personal control markedly less often than they practice those monitored by the breast center, even though the professional staff encourages breast self-exam, low-fat diet, exercise, and relaxation training. Thirty-nine percent of the women, however, judged relaxation training very helpful in coping with the anxiety and fear that accompany both regular mammograms and the occasional appearance of breast cysts requiring diagnosis and treatment. Significantly, only a minority experience daily anxiety and concern about their high-risk status; most report that these emotions arise at the times of scheduled exams, of treatments needed for a benign condition, or when a friend or relative develops breast cancer.

Group members felt that breast cancer bonds them to other women, especially to their mothers and sisters. Forty percent of the sample had both mothers and sisters diagnosed with breast cancer, 47 percent had mothers only, and 13 percent had sisters only. The attitudes of the health professionals treating her also help determine whether a woman can mobilize her own resources for effective coping. These professionals routinely confront the anger, anxiety, and despair that high-risk women feel. Optimal care requires respect for both a woman's genetic legacy and her feelings about it.

The Program for Successful Living presented in Part 4, chapters 9 through 12, was developed to help high-risk women gain a sense of effectiveness and personal control over their health and breast cancer. It grows out of the protocol used during the Georgetown University Comprehensive Breast Center study, which (1) examined attitudes toward and beliefs about health and breast cancer, (2) identified healthy and unhealthy ways of coping with the stress of daily living, (3) developed personally effective techniques of relaxation and stress management, and (4) included instruction and practice in risk-reducing strategies of breast self-exam, low-fat diet, and regular exercise.

This program of emotional support and medical care stands on a foundation of health behavior research that demonstrates the importance of an individual's belief in her ability to begin and successfully maintain strategies that promote health. Therefore, the suggested cognitive techniques help high-risk women understand their resistance to self-care while strengthening the skills and confidence they need to deal with their high-risk status. The program emphasizes that effective coping requires both the knowledge and conviction that one can take competent control of her own breast cancer risk.

The following guidelines for understanding a woman's cognitive, emotional, and behavioral responses emerged from the information gained in the focus groups:

1. The breast cancer experiences of other women in a high-risk woman's family contribute to her sense of personal vulnerability and her coping ability.

- A woman whose sister has had breast cancer feels particularly vulnerable, especially when the sister's breast cancer follows the mother's and there are now two immediate family members with the disease.
- The younger the woman when her mother died of breast cancer, the stronger the sense of personal loss and concern when she reaches the age at which her mother died. This concern extends to developing breast cancer and abandoning her own children, especially when they reach the age she was when her mother died.

2. The frequency, intensity, and duration of thinking about high-risk status indicate the level of threat and stress this situation is creating in a woman's life.

3. Eliciting a woman's emotional responses to high-risk status can help her mobilize her resources and coping abilities. Reduced stress and effective coping are correlated with increased willingness to practice health behaviors such as clinical breast exams, mammograms, breast self-exams, diet, exercise, and relaxation training.

4. Satisfying relationships with health professionals are critical for successful coping and well-being of high-risk women. Patient-professional relationships involving trust, mutual respect, and mutual decision making appear to be necessary and effective with this population.

The women who participated in the research project at the Georgetown University Comprehensive Breast Center contributed significantly to the insights and information in this book. They believed that the project could improve the quality of both their own lives and those of other women. Many felt they had found "true" sisters through this project; all felt supported and nurtured in their efforts to explore their unfinished thoughts and feelings about breast cancer. We salute their bravery and commitment and hope that this book merits their trust.

# *Acknowledgments*

MANY PEOPLE besides the authors contribute to the writing of a book. Since its inception three and one-half years ago, this project has benefited from ideas, support, and time generously given by a number of individuals. Dr. Sandra M. Swain, director of the Georgetown University Comprehensive Breast Center, welcomed this endeavor into the center and eagerly collaborated with, endorsed, and encouraged the focus groups and surveys. Kathleen Foster, R.N., nursing coordinator at the breast center, along with staff members Joy Dritschilo, R.N., and Janet Katyal, R.N., provided important assistance with patient contact and data collection. Kathleen's enthusiasm and her excellent instruction in breast self-exam were great motivators.

A number of people provided help crucial to completing the research in a timely fashion. Michael Kramer of the Video Services Department at Towson State University videotaped the focus groups, his sensitivity and expertise producing excellent recordings. Lisa DeGrouchy and Donna Gugel devoted many hours to data coding, analysis, and videotape transcription. Towson State University helped support the research through faculty research and development grants. The efforts of Dean Esslinger, Associate Dean of Faculty Development and Research, and Lynn Johnson, Director, Office of Research Administration, and their staffs are also greatly appreciated.

Companion focus groups were also conducted during the summer of 1990 in Charlotte, North Carolina, through the Mecklenburg County Health Department. This project gathered information on the health beliefs and practices of black, low-income women in relation to breast and cervical cancer. Susan Bacot and Priscilla Laula coordinated these groups, and their collaboration and support contributed significantly to this research.

A number of colleagues offered assistance through lengthy discussions. Drs. Sheryle Gallant and Gwendolyn Puryear Keita were always available to listen, make suggestions, and give encouragement. They share our commitment to furthering research in women's health. Drs. Jack Osman and Phyllis Ensor showed consistent—and much appreciated—support. Sandra Esslinger of the American Cancer Society gave generously of her time in helping to obtain materials used in preparing this book.

Very special thanks go to Barbara Lowenstein, our literary agent, for her help in conceptualizing this project, and to Janet Goldstein, our editor, and Peternelle van Arsdale, her assistant editor, for their guidance in shaping it and their patience in seeing it through to print.

Throughout months of writing, our families offered understanding and encouragement. Our husbands, Jeff Schaler and Jordan Benderly, and our children, Magda Schaler and Daniel and Alicia Benderly, have our thanks for tolerating the evenings and weekends of work. As editor of her high school paper, Magda showed a special understanding of deadlines!

We owe a great debt to the many women who participated in the research, devoting time and energy to completing surveys and sharing their insights and experiences. Their contribution was a gift of love to both the women in their families and the high-risk women everywhere who will benefit from this book.

And finally, we remember Marcia Ila Hafter, a dear friend of Renee's whose untimely death from breast cancer inspired a personal research interest in this crucial area of women's health.

*Challenging the
Breast Cancer
Legacy*

# INTRODUCTION

❧

# My Mother, My Sister, My Daughter, Myself

ABBY SPEAKS for many women. She may speak for you. "On a bad day, I figure I'm going to have to get it. Both my mother and my sister had it," she says of the anxiety that pervades her life.

"It" is breast cancer, a terror that tends to run in families. Her mother and her sister are only two of many thousands— 44,000 American women from their mid-twenties to their nineties died of breast cancer in 1991. Almost 175,000 more were newly diagnosed with this disease that is the largest killer of women in the prime of life. "On a good day," Abby goes on, "I figure I'm not much worse off than normal-risk women. But I think about it every day."

So do many of the millions who share her legacy. So, perhaps, do you.

Every American woman faces roughly one chance in nine of developing breast cancer at some point during her lifetime. But for the daughters, sisters, or mothers of those who actually get breast cancer, the odds may be two or even three times as high. Only advanced age and a previous bout of breast cancer

I

raise an individual's risk more than a close blood tie, particularly to an immediate relative who had cancer in both breasts.

But as Abby knows all too well, physical danger is only part of the wallop that this disease packs. Its emotional effects usually spread far beyond the patient, causing her sisters, daughters, and mother to go through difficult changes of their own. The futures of these still-healthy women may suddenly seem more constrained by the threat of illness or early death; their present more complicated by deep and conflicting feelings of anger, guilt, regret, hopelessness, and anxiety. Like many women, you may have found that your family's legacy of breast cancer adds a new, and perhaps frightening, dimension to what it means to belong to your particular clan; to be a daughter, sister, and mother; to pass that legacy on to daughters of your own. It may bring new anxiety about your own and your children's or potential children's futures.

But like many women, you may find it difficult to express or even acknowledge these emotions. Indeed, you may not even recognize their traces in the patterns of your life. Like many who have watched or cared for a mother or sister during her illness, you may have suppressed your own needs and emotions for the duration of the crisis. But for you, as for many women, these feelings may return years, even decades later—brought on perhaps by a friend's or relative's breast cancer, or by the need to have your own breast biopsied, or even by taking part in a research study.

## BREAKING SILENCE

Until very recently the special issues facing high-risk women remained largely hidden, both from the women themselves and from others. Medical and psychological researchers have long studied breast cancer patients, building a large literature about what happens, both emotionally and physically, as the disease progresses. But the patient's daughters, sisters, and mothers—who suddenly find themselves under a threat that many do not understand and cannot freely discuss—have received almost no systematic attention. Only in the last few years have high-risk but healthy relatives emerged as a group with distinct problems, issues, and reactions. And only in a handful of centers have researchers begun to study those concerns. This book reports on research that is pioneering the field.

If you have a family legacy of breast cancer, you know that, much as you love the kinswoman who was ill, your own concerns differ from hers and deserve separate attention. You will find that this book discusses *your* issues on your terms.

What kind of woman finds herself at high risk for breast cancer? Every kind of woman, from every racial and ethnic background, from every economic and social group, from every region and walk of life. She might be young or have reached a mature age; she might be single, married, or formerly married; she might or might not have children or grandchildren. She might have a sophisticated understanding of cancer or know very little about it.

You will meet, in the pages that follow, women who match all of these descriptions. What they have in common is a family legacy of breast cancer. But regardless of their backgrounds, interests, life situations, or levels of sophistication, their accounts describe some quite similar experiences and raise a number of similar issues.

Often, a woman's problems begin with the very way she learns about her unwelcome new status as a member of a high-risk group. First, she goes through the intense trauma of a loved one's illness. Only later—sometimes years later—does she focus on the fact that this difficult experience has troubling implications for herself. During the illness, her mother's or sister's needs seemed far greater and more immediate than her own. Alongside the ordeal of a loved one, thinking of her own future welfare may have seemed secondary, even selfish. In the face of a relative's need for affection, care, and support, considering her own jeopardy may have felt disloyal, almost like blaming the patient for the new risk her relatives face.

If you recognize any part of your own story here, you, like many caring women, may have subordinated your own confusion and apprehension to your relative's need for love, support, and optimism; to the grief at her death; or to the desire of surviving family members for you to be "strong" in the face of bereavement. You may well believe that even possessing these negative emotions marks you as frivolous, unloving, self-indulgent, selfish, morbid, or neurotic.

But as much as you try to ignore these feelings, you, like Abby, may find that they never quite go away. These feelings continue to reverberate long afterward as you struggle to integrate the unpleasant fact of high-risk status into your present life, your understanding of the past, your relationships, your image of yourself as a woman, your image of womanhood itself.

And like Abby, you may not fully recognize how large these feelings loom in your inner life, how they cloud your hopes for your future, how much they contribute to anxiety and unease. In your conscious mind, you may underestimate or entirely dismiss the influence that high-risk status has on your day-to-day welfare. But like Abby, you may be struggling to find ways to live constructively and hopefully in the face of an ambiguity that can threaten both your sense of self and your very life.

Anne, whose mother died when she was ten, also speaks for a multitude of high-risk women. "I have no sisters," she says, "but through breast cancer I feel a sisterhood with other women. It is something that we share."

This sisterhood now numbers in the millions. But if you

are at high risk, you may not have realized how many sisters you actually have. You may not yet have drawn strength from the very numbers of those who face the same issues you do.

In the pages that follow, you will find many stories you can use to put your own experiences and concerns into perspective. You may find, for example, that anxieties and conflicts that you thought belonged to you alone or to the small circle of your immediate family are in fact surprisingly common—even normal—among women at high risk.

## HOW TO USE THIS BOOK

We hope that this book will help you find your own way to positive, hopeful living. We believe it can help you explore your own experience by sharing in the experiences of others. It will bring you the voices of women who have felt deeply and thought hard about the inheritance you share with them. It will help you to understand how the legacy of breast cancer has influenced possibly unsuspected aspects of yourself and how its impact changes over the course of your lifetime. Finally, the book will guide you in developing a practical approach to living a full life in the shadow of uncertainty—an approach that includes both medical surveillance to minimize your risk and effective psychological techniques to maximize your emotional adjustment, sense of control, and personal effectiveness.

We have designed the book to provide the tools you need to clarify, simplify, improve, and preserve your life as a high-risk woman. To remain healthy, every high-risk woman must commit herself to a lifelong program of active steps to safeguard her health. These include regular mammograms, clinical breast exams, and self-exams, along with attention to diet and exercise. Such a commitment takes discipline, determination, and a clear understanding of the part each element plays.

But a person overwhelmed by negative emotions or trapped in unproductive reactions often cannot bring herself to start or maintain this potentially lifesaving program. Ironically, the terror and worry that she may develop breast cancer may keep her from doing all that she can to protect herself from the very fate she fears. That is why understanding your emotions concerning your relative's cancer and your own risk is vital to your own health. Only when you gain insight into your reactions can you also gain control over them; only when you have put your emotions into context can you put yourself in charge. Your choices and reactions, therefore, have a vital bearing on your future as a high-risk woman. And, like many people, you can learn to change reactions that stand in the way of your own true best interest.

That is why this book first helps you to understand your emotions and then teaches you to cope with them realistically and constructively. In Part 1, we begin by delving into family histories and personal memories, exploring, through the lives of many women, what your own legacy might mean to you. We will observe that individuals respond to this felt danger in profound, far-reaching, and complex, but—until now—little-recognized ways. We begin by exploring the experience of watching breast cancer develop in one's mother, both during childhood and in adulthood. These chapters concentrate on the issues raised when only one family member has been stricken. Next we consider the issues that arise when a sister gets cancer. This chapter also discusses the issues involved when multiple family members get breast cancer. All these chapters may not immediately relate to your own experience, but we hope that you will read all three nonetheless. Each contains insights relevant to all high-risk women that do not appear in other chapters. Together they give a broad yet detailed view.

Using these chapters as a basis for thinking about your

own story, you will see how age and stage of life have powerfully shaped your reactions. We will explain, for example, why the particular point in your life when the threat of breast cancer first arose strongly molds its meaning for you. And you will see how that meaning evolves through the stages of your own lifetime.

In Part 2, we'll explain the nature of cancer and the nature of risk. We'll show why the risk you face may be smaller than you thought. You'll see that high-risk status is not a uniform state but varies with each individual's family history and way of life. High risk, therefore, is not a sentence to be inevitably fulfilled but a mathematical probability that may or may not come to pass—in other words, not a fate but a figure of speech.

In Part 3, we will show you that you are not powerless in the face of this threat. You will see how your choices can influence the objective risk you face and, more importantly, how they can help determine the quality of your life. In Part 4, we will outline a practical plan that empowers you to live positively with the ambiguity inherent in your situation. We will explain in detail how you can reduce anxiety, depression, and fear and increase your peace of mind while doing all that is possible to minimize your risk.

The chapters that follow recount many personal experiences in the words of the people who lived them. We hope they will provide a beginning place for thinking about your own experiences—for comparing your feelings to those of the women in our pages, for considering which of the conclusions that we draw may apply to you. But you may find some of these tales uncomfortable, even painful—too familiar, too close to your own bone. You, like many others, may have long ago buried the memories of a relative's—especially a mother's—suffering. The accounts you will read may stir up incidents or feelings that you had consigned to the depths of your unconscious.

For example, after Jeannette, now in her sixties, had spent some time trying to recall her mother's long-ago cancer she admitted, "I didn't realize how much I had blocked out about my mother's death in 1955. Until I started trying to remember again, I had forgotten that I had terrible nightmares for three years afterward."

Something similar happened to Anne. During the time that she was trying to recall her family's experiences, she felt "very, very tired. And I knew it wasn't from working too hard or being sick. I almost decided not to continue trying to remember.

"But," she goes on, smiling, "obviously I did. I felt I had to tell my experience—for myself, for all women, for my mother."

Exploring your feelings about the cancer of women close to you will permit insight both into your reactions during that stressful time and into the methods you used to cope both then and since. Many women who undertake this journey find it deeply liberating, freeing them to take positive action, to experience themselves as less alone, less helpless, more whole.

We hope that the same may happen for you.

# I

❦

## *Understanding the Family Legacy*

# 1

❦

# *Losing Mother Early*

I DIED when I was ten," Anne once told a close friend. "I don't remember saying it," she recalls later with a solemn laugh. "I meant to say—I thought I had said, 'My *mother* died when I was ten.' But my friend insisted, 'No, that's not what you said. It was one of the first things you ever told me about yourself. I made a special note of it.' "

Anne's own evolving sense of life's goodness and promise, the optimism and security that should accompany youth, perished, she now sees, in her mother's losing fight for life. The adult Anne has spent decades struggling to understand and heal the hurt done by her mother's illness and death. Now nearing fifty, she knows that whatever else has happened or will happen in her lifetime, that shock is its central emotional incident. It riddled the bedrock of her psyche with cracks and faults that only later became visible, as she tried to establish her own self-image and relationships.

Perhaps you recognize your own early life in Anne's feelings. In this chapter we will concentrate on the reactions of daughters who were children younger than the age of puberty when their mothers confronted breast cancer. The outcome of that struggle, whether the mother survived or succumbed, often has a profound and lasting effect on a girl's entire life.

Our research shows, in fact, that women who remember losing their mothers to breast cancer while they were still children tend to suffer the deepest and most pervasive psychological effects both from that loss and from their own high-risk status. But as we'll see later in this chapter, girls whose mothers fought breast cancer and recovered tend to suffer much less damage and to develop differently.

## GROWING UP WITH BREAST CANCER

Central to the early loss of one's mother is the fact that a child lacks a fully developed sense of herself. "I think that suffering through this when you're so young," says Harriet, who lost her mother to breast cancer at eleven, "has a tremendous impact. If you're a child, and you suffer such a great loss, you don't really understand it. You're never allowed to grieve over it. You never really get over it. It's bound to give you a special perspective on breast cancer."

And indeed, our research bears Harriet out. For daughters who suffered such a shattering blow during the early years of their own emotional development, breast cancer—both their mothers' deaths and their own vulnerability to the disease—becomes a *developmental issue* in their own lives, an issue that recurs in various forms during the life course. The emotions surrounding it remain unresolved—and for many, unresolvable—throughout their lives.

For these women, the anxiety, vulnerability, and dread experienced in childhood often return quite strongly at the anniversary of the mother's death, even long afterward. Yvonne, for example, now in her twenties, lost her mother when she was ten. She felt forced to assume the responsibility of cooking and cleaning for the family. Every year she finds the anniversary of her mother's death extremely painful—much more so, she believes, than do her father or her brothers. "Time hasn't worked for me to get over it," she says. "You keep wanting to talk to your mom about dating and things like that."

Her grandmother's death from breast cancer a few years later only sharpened her fear of the disease that seems able to take all the important women in her life. She knows keenly that she has not healed from her early sorrows. Now, as an adult, she has resolved to seek counseling and support to begin that process.

And distress can mount even higher as the daughter passes two crucial points in her own adult life: when she reaches the age at which her mother died and when her own child approaches the age at which she witnessed the death. At either of these milestones, many people, including Anne and Harriet, find their distress so severe that they feel they must try to find new ways of managing it. For many, the answer is taking active steps to seek preventive care.

But much less obvious effects also wait to ambush the daughter as she tries to achieve such critical emotional passages as becoming a woman and becoming a mother. Both the fact of the mother's death and its specific cause—breast cancer—have significant and lasting repercussions for the daughter's relationship to her own body and to the people around her. *Understanding the hidden source of her feelings can help her separate the reality of her present situation from the unalterable tragedy of the past.*

For Anne, her mother's suffering remains close, personal, and ever-threatening. "I myself have had breast lumps twice," she tells a group of women gathered for one of our focus groups. "They needed to be biopsied and I was absolutely terrified. Fortunately, both of them turned out to be harmless cysts. But during the time I was waiting for the results, all the memories of my mother's illness came back. All the screaming and pain came back."

Abby, motherless since the age of thirteen, releases a sigh. "The worst part of the whole thing was being there to witness the suffering, the wasting away."

For many girls, though, this pain had no outlet. "I come from a family of deniers," Anne tells the other women matter-of-factly. "The illness, the possibility of death, were not discussed. All the time my mother was sick, they didn't really level with me about what was going on or what would happen. No one told me then that that my mother had cancer, that she was going to die. She was on her deathbed, they had nurses in the house, and they were telling us that she would get well. They didn't tell me anything until one day they suddenly told me she was dying. And after she did die, the very next day after, I went to school as usual, as if nothing had happened. The teacher said, 'Anne, I'm surprised to see you today.' But I said, just so flippantly"—and here she gives her head the same snippy toss she remembers from so long ago— " 'Well, it's a school day, isn't it?'

"In our family it was business as usual. My father farmed us out to relatives and didn't speak of my mother's illness again. He died just last year, and he never talked to me about it. It left me with a great deal of anger toward him."

Harriet has been listening closely. Now she takes a deep breath. "I was eleven when my mother died. I knew that she was sick, but I never knew with what. And I was never allowed to grieve. I never even knew she had breast cancer, not until I was in college. They kept that from me, the way they did in those days. I guess they wanted to protect me, but in fact the way they did it made me feel responsible for her death. My aunts used to say to my brothers and me, 'Play quietly so your mother can get better, be good so your mother can get well.'

And when of course she didn't, it was terrible for us. Was it because we didn't play quietly enough, weren't good enough?"

"They told me she would get better," Abby says. "They also shielded me. They wanted to protect me. It was a great disservice."

She pauses and looks closely at Harriet and Anne, whom she met only a week ago. Then she speaks in a low, almost reluctant voice: "After your mothers died," she asks, "did your fathers sort of check out emotionally? Did they just sort of leave you? Not connect with you? Not pay you any real attention?"

Harriet and Anne nod.

"My father just checked out after my mother died," Abby repeats. "In a way that was almost worse than my mother's death. He was there, but he just didn't function. He sort of disconnected from the family."

"Then he remarried," says Anne. "I guess it's sort of a normal reaction."

"My stepmother legally adopted me," Harriet says, "and then abandoned me after my father died."

Says Abby, "My brother was away at college and I was left with housekeepers. It was like being abandoned twice."

The word "abandoned" hangs in the air. Three or four decades afterward, for these women approaching or well into midlife, a mother's death from breast cancer still feels like willful desertion, a father's remarriage like a betrayal. In their deepest feelings, these grown women, mothers themselves, sometimes still feel like motherless children.

Feelings of abandonment, grief, and yearning to be cared for commonly plague children during a parent's cancer, found a study sponsored by the National Cancer Foundation.[1] Even when the parent survives, youngsters angrily resent being excluded from the circle of care. Another study, by Rosenfeld and colleagues, also documented that adolescent daughters feel inadequate support during the crisis of a mother's mastectomy.[2] This research, along with our own, highlights the need for families to include children in some meaningful way in the experience of serious disease.[3] Those who participate with understanding in a parent's terminal illness suffer less anxiety than those who do not. And this inclusion may have a protective effect, especially for girls who lose their mothers to illness early in life and become prone to lifelong depression.[4]

## BECOMING A WOMAN

In Harriet, Abby, Anne, and Yvonne's families, the mother's breast cancer had become a nonsubject, if not taboo then certainly ignored. But the daughters had to express their feelings at some point, and finally each of these four did. Significantly, this happened most intensely as they tried to negotiate, without a mother's guidance, the passage to womanhood.

"I didn't know my mother had had cancer for a long time," Anne says. "My cousin told me after I finished high school. And I remember being terrified. I have a clear recollection of standing in front of my mirror and feeling my bones here"—her hand moves across her upper chest—"and thinking, 'Lumps! Lumps! Lumps everywhere!'

"I lost a lot of weight," she continues. I was terrified of getting fat. I just stopped eating. People kept asking me if I had been sick. But I thought I looked great. I was convinced I was svelte. Any weight gain would terrify me, even the very thought of getting fat. I was really paranoid about fat. I dieted so hard that my periods stopped. I was afraid to tell anyone that they had for fear they'd think I was pregnant, which was the cardinal sin in my family. The doctors thought I had thyroid problems that were emotionally related."

Harriet nods in recognition. "First my mother died, and then when I was seventeen, my father died too. I was sent to live with an aunt. About that time, my periods just stopped for nearly three years. And I was also dieting very hard then, exercising all the time. I was on the verge of anorexia. My aunt got worried and sent me to specialists. For a while they thought I had a pituitary tumor. Finally, a physician told me that he thought my problem was that I was suppressing everything, holding everything in. It was all just too much for me and I guess in a way I broke down. In my body, everything just stopped. Finally, I realized that living with my aunt was not any good for me. I realized that there was something really wrong with the whole situation and with me. I moved away and got an apartment with a girlfriend. I think I should probably have gone into therapy, but I didn't. Then gradually I got better."

Abby solemnly admits that, though her slenderness never approached the terminal state of anorexia, she has felt a lifelong "terror of gaining weight" and compulsion to keep it off.

But why assume that these problems belong to the emotional legacy of breast cancer? Why draw any developmental connection between childhood trauma and young adult anxiety? Most young women worry about their weight. Many with living, healthy mothers suffer anorexia and eating disorders.

But in their abnormal alarm at normal weight gain, in the stark symbolism of their fear of flesh, Anne, Harriet, and Abby are typical of many high-risk women. They were struggling to understand their mothers' fate at the same time they were becoming women themselves.

"Because of what had happened to my mother," Anne explains, "I connected being a woman with dying of cancer. If I became a woman like her, if I gained weight, if I filled out, if I had breasts, I'd die. I remember not wanting to be a woman. So, by not eating, I made myself shrink back to being a child, to what I remember as a happier time."

Every daughter incorporates her mother's example into her own identity, her vision of womanhood and of herself as a woman. But Abby, Anne, and Harriet had a terrifying example. Womanhood meant dying a painful and uniquely womanly death, a death that began in the most womanly of organs. No task is more central to childhood and adolescence than building a firm sense of self, ideally with the help, and partly in the image, of a loving mother. But if her mother dies when this task has scarcely begun, the daughter, deprived of her model and guide, may not succeed in building a rounded picture of her mother's life or of her own possibilities as a woman.

Of course, it's true that no daughter can know her mother's life in its entirety. Have you heard the old joke about a daughter who complains when her mother does something apparently out of character?

"That's not like you, Mom."

"How do you know that?"

"I know you. I've known you all my life."

"Yes, dear, but you haven't known me all of *my* life."

In the sweep of a mother's entire lifetime, her cancer constitutes a relatively brief, final episode, utterly divorced from the loves, friendships, work, and accomplishments that defined her personhood. For the grieving girl, though, the part she sees as most salient—the illness and death—becomes a central meaning of that life.

*And so, a daughter may express the fear of her mother's fate by attempting not to be like her, by struggling to forestall her own change from girl into woman.*

Normally, this change happens over a period of years, as a girl's body gradually becomes a woman's. The first manifestation is a speeding up of growth, both in height and weight. For most girls, these changes, though perhaps confusing, bring promise of the excitement of the teen years and adulthood. For high-risk daughters, the physical signs of oncoming womanhood can seem to foretell an inevitable doom. Keeping off curves and ceasing to menstruate—erasing the outward signs of what threatens to happen to them—became a means to prevent their mothers' fate from becoming their own.

Excessive fear of gaining weight in young womanhood, which can sometimes become quite severe, appears to afflict many women who lost their mothers to breast cancer before their own adolescence. It is an attempt not to become women like their mothers. At the time, however, many of these women do not make a conscious connection between their own condition and their mothers' illness.

And, indeed, Anne and Harriet, in starving themselves and stopping their periods, had hit upon both a symbolic and a physiological truth, a connection between fat and femaleness that is far more than metaphoric. The spurt in weight that precedes female puberty is no coincidence, but rather a physiological necessity. The average girl leaves childhood as lean as a boy. When she emerges from puberty several years later, a healthy woman carries twice the body fat of a man of comparable height; rapid weight gain is often a necessary precondition both to womanhood and to womanly reproductive function.

The human body doesn't even permit menstruation to begin until a girl carries certain absolute and relative quantities of fat. Youngsters who don't build up those reserves—child ballerinas or Olympic swimming and gymnastic hopefuls, for example—menstruate years later than less active agemates. Sedentary girls who build up fat reserves early tend to menstruate correspondingly earlier. And older women can also starve their periods to a halt, as happened, for example, to inmates in Nazi concentration camps.

So grieving young girls, by the same tactic of starvation, were able to hold off for a while at least the dreaded reality of womanhood. But ultimately, of course, they could not prevent but only delay the physical inevitability of womanhood.

## WILL I BECOME MY MOTHER?

With that step into womanhood, they lay themselves open to the next developmental issue relating to breast cancer. Getting married forces women to consider pregnancy, another decision that would tie them even more closely to their mothers' fates. Should they become mothers themselves?

Women who lost their mothers in childhood often feel that having children of their own identifies them very closely with their own mothers and thus presages their own deaths by breast cancer. They may experience intense anxiety during pregnancy and before they or their children reach ages symbolically connected with their mothers' illness or death.

"I'm really very fatalistic about the whole thing," Abby says. "I'm convinced it's only a matter of time before I get it. For a long time I refused to have children. But my husband said, 'If you don't I'll divorce you,' so in the end I went ahead and had them. That made it worse. It's not that I regret having children. I have wonderful children. I'd never say that I regret having children, but having them made my fear worse."

For Anne, the initial decision to conceive was not a struggle. But her body once again spoke for her, emotionally rejecting her own conscious choice. And the pain of identification with her mother ultimately became all the more concrete. "My mother got breast cancer at thirty-four, soon after my youngest brother's birth. She died ten years later, at forty-three. I had thought for a long time that the pregnancy had brought on the cancer. So when I became pregnant myself, I became terrified that my pregnancy would lead to cancer, just the way hers had. I believed that as soon as I had my baby, I would die. I became intensely anxious. I was anxious throughout the pregnancy." A perfectly normal, trouble-free pregnancy—one that, in other circumstances, Anne could have enjoyed—became instead nine months of dread.

Anne remained healthy after the birth, however. The feared postpartum cancer did not develop. But then, when her daughter was about seven, her anxiety had begun to build anew. In her mind, she was approaching another target date for cancer. "I worked out how old I was when my mother died—the year, the month, and the day. And also how old my mother was. I became convinced that I would die when I reached the same age my mother was when she died." But she reached and passed that age without incident.

As her daughter advanced through the elementary grades, though, Anne felt her terror returning. "Then I started to believe that I'd die when my daughter reached the age *I* was when my mother died."

Harriet concurs. "My mother died when I was eleven. I've been getting more and more afraid that when my daughter reaches that age, I'll get breast cancer and it will metastasize and I'll die the way my mother did. My daughter is now ten and a half. I find myself getting very anxious."

For Anne at least, that milestone also came and went without mishap. Only after surviving two dreaded dates has she come to believe that her life is not destined to recapitulate her mother's, that she is free to live a life of her own.

## FEARING FOR OUR CHILDREN

Pregnancy usually ends in birth, which presents the mother with a growing child, an emissary of the future, a proxy for herself, and an utterly helpless dependent. Now the developmental dread can attach itself to a new innocent. Seeing themselves as mothers likely to succumb to breast cancer, these women see their daughters as the next generation likely to inherit high-risk status. Abby has sons. Anne and Harriet, though, have long worried about passing their family's genetic propensity on to daughters. Yvonne always assumed, because her mother died young of breast cancer, that she would be unwise to have children herself. An aunt, who watched not only a sister (Yvonne's mother) but her own mother die of breast cancer, came to a similar conclusion. Now childless and postmenopausal, the older woman regrets her decision and wants Yvonne to avoid the same mistake.

But Anne, Abby, and Harriet fear that they may pass on more than the possibility of getting cancer. Just as they see themselves recapitulating their mothers' lives, they see their children possibly recapitulating their own. Just as they identify with their mothers as women who had cancer, they identify with their sons and daughters as children of such threatened women.

"I didn't want to have children," Abby says, "because I didn't want to leave them as I had been left. I know how I suffered, and I don't want them to suffer that way." Now that she has sons, this possibility weighs heavily on her. "Before I had children, it was just me. I was only responsible for myself. What happened didn't matter as much as it does now. But now, I have them and I feel a tremendous responsibility to them. It has made my fear much worse."

None of Abby's sons has reached age thirteen, the threshold to her orphanhood. Perhaps when they do, or when, in a few years, she outlives her mother's age of death, her anxiety may abate somewhat. But her sons may have to reach adulthood—and she a stage of life that her mother never attained—before her mother's illness loses its hold on Abby's future.

## IN SUMMARY

A girl who loses her mother to breast cancer before she herself has reached puberty suffers a trauma that *can* transform breast cancer into a developmental issue. She can expect the emotions surrounding her mother's death to reemerge at points during her life when she is concerned with the issues of her own health or womanhood. This often happens during such periods of transition as:

- Puberty or adolescence—the passage from girlhood to womanhood.
- Pregnancy or childbirth—the passage to motherhood.
- A child reaching the age she was when her mother died—the memory of her own vulnerability and loss.
- Reaching the age at which her mother died—another form of passage to a life stage beyond what her mother attained.
- Being reminded of her genetic vulnerability—finding a breast lump or having a problematic mammogram, or a close woman relative having a breast procedure or a diagnosis of breast cancer.

And what of the woman who, as a child, saw her mother fight breast cancer and win?

"I was a little girl when my mother had her cancer," Phyllis says. "I knew almost nothing about it. I knew my mother was sick, but my father denied it was cancer. No one spoke of cancer in those days. I believe she had X-ray treatment. I know she was ill for a very long time, but she got better. She died twenty years later of heart disease. My mother was fat and always feared losing weight because it was a sign of cancer. But she coped, and she was a great coper. She just slogged on."

For Phyllis, the traumatic time of her mother's illness ended before she was even aware of its possible consequences. Cancer did not darken her childhood; her mother was sick for a while but then recovered. For her and women like her, breast cancer is not a developmental issue tied to the nature of one's own womanhood. Rather, it is a genetic risk that causes concern. That's why women who understand and acknowledge their risk often take advantage of the early detection strategies that can preserve their health. We'll discuss these in detail in parts 2 and 3.

Childhood memories of a mother's breast cancer cause deep and pervasive consequences. Most breast cancers, however, occur after menopause, when daughters generally have grown up. These daughters face their own set of issues regarding breast cancer. It is to them that we turn next.

# 2

❦

# *Cancer Come Lately*

W HEN MY mother was diagnosed with breast cancer," Lilian says, "I was married, living in a city far away from my parents, and pregnant with my third child. By the time she was in the last stages of her illness, I had three children under five. I was nursing a baby. I couldn't really take any part in caring for her. She had my father, and a strong support network in our hometown.

"I loved my mother very much, but I had no doubt where my responsibility lay: taking care of my own large, young family. She understood why I couldn't get to see her very much. She understood that I had no choice but to take care of my responsibilities at home. I was nursing a baby all through the time of her dying, at the funeral and everything. I knew it wouldn't do anyone any good for me to wear myself out. I had to keep myself healthy, both physically and psychologically, for my children. I just had to be positive."

As her mother lay dying, Linda had a different idea. "For the last month of my mother's life, I lived with her, essentially in the same room with her. When she became terribly sick, she was living down south and I was living here, a thousand miles away. For those weeks, I was there with her almost all the time, to see that the room, the nurses, everything was all right. I'm not a nurse, but I did do a lot of caring for her. It was a great strain but I wouldn't have had it any other way. It was hard on my own family, but I have a wonderful, supportive husband. He took care of our three kids through that whole terrible time. And I think it really affected my youngest son. He was one and a half at that time, and since then he's had trouble with separation. I think it must go back to that time. I've read a lot of child development books and I see that that's a bad time in a child's development for his mother to be away. Still, I did what I thought was for the best, what I had to. As I said, I wouldn't have had it any other way."

During her mother's final illness, Teresa lived nearby. "My mother had breast cancer for eight years. She was fifty-three when she died. [Teresa was then in her late twenties.] I think that when the cancer came back and she found out she was dying, her biggest concern was with her kids, with how it would affect us. She was at a major oncology department, so we were always confident she was getting the best care. She didn't like to talk about any of it. Mothers don't want you to be all upset. We wanted to talk about it, but she didn't. She had four girls and we may very well be in the same seat some-day. She tried to suppress it.

"After I accepted in my heart that my mother was going to die, I thought that the most important thing was to let her know that we loved her. I'd call her up and if she didn't feel like talking, I'd say, 'I just want to listen to you breathe. When you get tired, just hang up the phone.' Or I'd go visit her and lie on the bed with her and she could reach over and hold my hand if she wanted to.

"My sisters were all basket cases. I'm the oldest. Maybe that's why I didn't fall apart emotionally. I and one other sister stayed in close touch with the doctor. The fact that I didn't get all upset doesn't mean that I didn't care as much as they did.

Of course I did. But it's just another thing that's been sent to us. You've got to deal with it. You've got to not dwell on it. You've got to go on."

For Laura, her mother's final illness meant undertaking a supreme labor of love. "When my mother was done with her last treatments in the hospital, the doctor said she was too sick to go home. He said she had to go to a nursing home. But she really didn't want to do that. She started to cry. My father didn't want her to, either, but after she regained her composure, he said, 'Well, if that's what the doctor says, I guess we'll have to do it.' My mother was very unhappy about this. She didn't say so, but I knew anyway. She didn't say anything after that because she thought it would be easier for us and we wanted her to go. She didn't want us to have a lot of trouble. And the doctor was sure that we couldn't care for her at home. I had a baby and I was working full-time and my brother was off working.

"But I said, 'No, we're not going to do that. We're not sending her to any nursing home. We're taking her home.' So then I had to find out how to take care of her. In the end, I was surprised that it wasn't as hard to do as I thought it would be. I was able to arrange for hospice care at home. What really made me angry was that the doctor made absolutely no effort to help us.

"But we made it work. It worked out beautifully. I think my mom was really grateful. I took a leave from my job. In the end, it was only a matter of two months. The visiting nurses would come to see her, and we also had nurse's aides with her for sixteen hours a day. I was there for the other eight hours. My mother was very content with this arrangement and it was, in spite of all that was happening to her, a wonderful time. One thing that made it especially wonderful was that she wanted to write letters to all her friends about what they had meant to her. Of course, she couldn't write, but she dictated all the letters to me and I wrote them, crying a lot. She wrote to people we had never even heard of, people she had known in high school! Everyone wrote back wonderful letters, saying what she had meant to them, how she had influenced their lives. It showed her the great effect she had had on people. It also meant a great deal to us to get all those letters. I really think people should do more things like this, because it lets people see the effect they had on others."

Four daughters, four mothers, four very different families. If you were an adult when your mother developed breast cancer, you may recognize yourself and your family in one or more of these experiences. Or perhaps not; families handle this crisis in many different ways, and yours may have found yet a different one, more suited to your own circumstances.

Still, a single conclusion strikingly emerges from the many stories that women told us, and probably from your own as well: Women who are adults during their mothers' breast cancer have reactions and perspectives very different from those of women who experience their mothers' breast cancer as children.

A mother's cancer is almost always a shattering emotional blow—to her adult daughters, to her husband, to everyone in the family. The psychologists Rosemary Lichtman and Shelley Taylor and their colleagues found, in fact, that it can often disrupt the relationship between mother and daughter.[1] And the worse the mother's prognosis or her psychological adjustment to the disease, the worse the disruption may be. Both adolescent and postadolescent daughters, their research found, were distressed by fear of the legacy and by their mothers' demands for emotional support. In fact, the mother's fear of mutilation by mastectomy, of losing femininity, of needing further treatment, and of dying probably exacerbated the daughter's fear.

Despite these traumatic times, however, once the crisis passes, it usually does not have the kind of deep, long-lasting emotional effects on grown daughters that it can have on children. For adult daughters it generally does not become a central issue in their own emotional lives. They don't usually experience distress that reemerges repeatedly throughout their adult years. This is not to deny that a mother's death at any age can be a major emotional trauma. Linda, for example, had a severe grief reaction—"cancer phobia" and anxiety attacks that struck her frequently for almost two years. But her grieving finally ended and did not leave her with any lingering psychological problems. The difference is not in the degree of grief—this varies among individuals and is deeply personal—but the fact that childhood loss usually has lifelong emotional effects, while adult loss usually does not.

## FACING THE CHALLENGE

The grown daughter's circumstances are useful in understanding the form that her reaction takes.

*As a daughter's own life evolves, so does her understanding of and role in her mother's illness.* In early adulthood, she probably doesn't view herself as her mother's caretaker, and her mother may not accept her in that role. Jane, for example, found that her mother got along well without much help. "I didn't feel there was very much I could do," she says. "I was far away when she had her operation. And she got over that fairly quickly and is fine now. All I could do was call on the phone a lot."

But as caring for others grows to be part of the daughter's own identity, and as the mother comes to accept her as more of an equal adult, some daughters may also adopt a helper's role in the mother's illness.

Eleanor's mother had two bouts of cancer. Eleanor found

herself playing very different roles in them. "I feel very guilty," she says now, more than a decade after her mother's death, "that when my mother first had cancer, I wasn't there. Looking back, it even surprises me how little I know of that first illness. I was young, recently married, all engrossed in my own life. And my father is a doctor, an old-style, authoritarian doctor. It was only when she was dying seven years later of metastases that I really became involved."

The same was true for Linda. "When she first got it, I was also young, just married, all wrapped up in that. Cancer really didn't mean much to me. I didn't really understand what it meant or could mean. I only did later, when it recurred."

For some daughters, however, a helper's role may not be appropriate. They may feel too upset, as did Teresa's sisters, or too angry over their mothers' cancer to play an active role in the illness. Or their relation with mother may be a difficult or distant one not based on caring and nurturing.

Daughters who do become caretakers, however, try to use their own adult strengths to strengthen the mother's coping skills—and, incidentally, to insulate themselves from the kind of psychic damage suffered by younger daughters. A number of adult resources allow a grown daughter to become her mother's helper or even caretaker.

### Selfhood and Personhood

First among the strengths of an adult is a solid sense of self. Vulnerability to breast cancer looms large in the personal identities of young girls who watch their mothers die. Their mothers' illness and death is a vital fact about *themselves,* a deep and troublesome part of their sense of who they are as women and as human beings. But a daughter who faces her mother's illness as an adult faces it with both the resources of independence and a much more independent sense of self. She has more effectively separated her own identity from her mother's. Her mother's fate concerns her but need not define her own fate.

"When I was a child," Eleanor recalls, "I would hold my hand next to my mother's and compare them. They were very similar. I liked that; I said I wanted to be just like her. But she didn't want me to say that. She was afraid I'd think that everything that happened to her would happen to me, that I would feel predestined to follow her path. She didn't want that. She wanted me to see myself as separate from her, as living my own life."

An adult daughter has worked at separating herself from the flesh-and-blood person who is her mother; she sees herself as a distinct individual with a distinct future. She sees her mother's cancer as belonging to mother, not necessarily to herself. Eve expresses her separateness from her mother by considering her family tree. "I sometimes think I look a lot more like my father's family than my mother's," she says. "I'm aware of the differences between me and my mother's family. Is this denial? I don't think so. But there always are two sides to the question of inheritance. When breast cancer is an issue, you're pushing and you're pulling between wanting and not wanting to be like your mother."

## Knowing the Score

An adult daughter watching her mother's cancer also has the advantage of knowing the details of the disease. It generally doesn't become a mystery or secret because parents rarely "protect" grown children from the seriousness of the cancer. As recently as two decades ago, in fact, it was family members who conspired with doctors to "protect" the terminally ill patient from knowing the true prognosis. Many adult daughters know a great deal about the medical, financial, emotional, and familial aspects of their mothers' disease, sometimes even more than the mothers themselves. And this prevents the disease from becoming a mystery or taboo, as it was for Abby, Anne, and Harriet.

Judy, for example, tells with pride the story of her mother's diagnosis. "My mother discovered her own breast cancer one day while she was sitting in the tub. She looked down and just saw a lump protruding from her breast. I'll never understand how she was able to do that. But she knew exactly what it was and what she had to do about it. She said that once she had seen it, it was like God had taken her by the hand and told her to get to the hospital."

Glenda can also recount the incident in detail. "My mother's cancer was discovered more or less by accident. She was going into the hospital for some minor surgery on something else. She said to the doctor, 'As long as I'm here, I might as well show you this.' Well, they got all excited and canceled the other surgery and got ready to operate on this right away. My father was out of town on business. He flew right back. By the time he got home the next day, she was recovering from surgery."

## Understanding of Life Cycle

What are the features that distinguish a daughter from her mother? The first answer is age: the fact that they belong to different generations, that the mother is mature while the daughter is young, that the mother is nearing or has completed menopause while the daughter is at another stage of life entirely. And the daughter's adult understanding of the seasons of life is a resource that allows her to put the illness in some sort of context.

Women whose mothers had cancer late in life, especially postmenopausally, often see it as a feature of aging, not as an inherent feature of womanhood. "My mother developed breast cancer a few years ago," says Jane. "I know that when that happens, it's supposed to make it more likely that you will, too. I do come to the breast center for checkups because that's the sensible thing to do, but I'm not really worried about myself right now. At thirty-six, I'm not yet feeling urgent about it. I feel that when I'm fifty, I'll be more concerned about it. But right now, I just take care of myself in the spirit of being responsible."

And Lee says, "Ever since my mother's cancer, I've been pretty concerned about myself, especially when they found some calcifications [often associated with cancer] in my mammogram. But then the doctor said that my mother's age when she got breast cancer, seventy-nine, reduced my own risk."

## Long-Distance Caring

What else separates the generations now? In more and more American families, the single greatest separator is distance. These days, a grown daughter probably doesn't live in her mother's house, perhaps not even in the same state or region of the country. Unless she makes a special effort to be constantly present, she may be much less involved in day-to-day developments like the details of feeding and nursing and hour-by-hour suffering, than a child living in the family house.

But being away also keeps the daughter from the emotional reality of the mother's experience, be it recovery from mastectomy, chemotherapy, and radiation or relapse and decline. "My mother recovered emotionally from her mastectomy very quickly," says Jane. "She made much faster progress than I expected. It's a year now, and being away, I'm still holding my breath even though she is already feeling much better. When I saw her after a couple of months, she was so much better than she was right after the operation that I was really surprised."

Judy's experience was similar. "Actually, her attitude was much better than mine. She is just fine. She was fifty-nine or sixty at the time of her diagnosis and mastectomy. I was in shock. My father was devastated. It was the first serious illness in the family. I thought everything would change, but when I spoke with her on the phone afterward, she sounded fine."

A body of research bears out these experiences. For breast cancer patients who were physically and psychologically healthy and not depressed before the disease struck, complete return to work and family activities generally takes a year or two at most.[2,3,4,5,6,7] In other words, cancers that do not recur generally have no long-lasting effects.

## A CALL TO ACTION

*Whether she is near or far, a grown daughter usually feels the need to take concrete steps to help her mother or parents cope.* She doesn't "play quietly so that mother can get better." Rather, many women take action to see that mother gets the best possible care. That's because one of the things that sharply distinguishes the generations is attitude.

"My mother's of a generation that doesn't question doctors," Roslyn says. "She just does what they say. But I thought she should have a second opinion. It bothered me that she didn't. I made lots of calls."

So did Ginnie. "My mother didn't want to bother with a second opinion either. She just accepted the treatment the doctor suggested. I wanted to make sure it was the right thing, the thing that would give her the best chance. I called around to experts in her particular cancer at different major centers— Sloan-Kettering, Johns Hopkins, Mayo. I just called them up out of the blue and explained the situation. I was actually quite surprised at how willing they were to talk to me and answer my questions. They thought that for her kind of tumor and number of nodes, the treatment she was getting was probably as good as anything."

But mother may not always appreciate or avail herself of a daughter's help. Roslyn recounts a particularly disturbing example.

"After my mother's mastectomy, I asked whether she was having chemo or anything," she recalls. "According to her, the doctor said that with only three nodes involved, she didn't need it. He said that three nodes or less didn't need anything beyond surgery.

"I knew that was wrong. I knew that with any nodes, you need some kind of follow-up treatment. But my parents wouldn't listen to me when I said that with any nodes you need something. I had done some research about it. They were living in Florida and there wasn't any really good hospital nearby. I said, 'Go down to Miami, go to the university medical center. Ask them there about the nodes.' But they wouldn't go. Miami's about two hours from where they live. They said they didn't want to drive that far! Can you imagine!

"Later, when the cancer came back, I told them that they ought to consider taking legal action, but they wouldn't listen to that either. I knew what the doctor told her was wrong, but they wouldn't listen."

## FAMILY TIES

As Roslyn's experience shows, *the drama of breast cancer plays itself out on the stage of existing family relationships.* Personalities don't change and strife doesn't vanish simply because someone falls ill. If anything, the stress of illness often sharpens conflict.

Roslyn's extended family, for example, had already begun to grapple with issues that are common as aging parents grow less able to cope on their own. Believing that her mother and father needed more care and showed less competence than in the past, she had begun to act a bit like their caretaker—a change that they resisted. She perceived her parents' refusal to drive an extra hour or two to get better medical care as the unreasonable stubbornness of old age, a sign of fading powers. But Mom and Dad may see her insistence that they go to an unfamiliar city for a consultation with an unknown doctor as an unwarranted intrusion into lives they had always managed on their own. In this family, an active middle-aged daughter at the height of her powers has already begun to threaten declining parents who feel their own powers ebbing away.

Ginnie's family also played old parent-child themes in the new key of cancer. "My middle sister has always had a very conflicted relationship with my mother," Ginnie says. "She says she had a miserable childhood, even though none of the rest of us remember her as being all that miserable. We were fairly poor, but she insists we were much richer than we were. She seems to feel that she didn't get what she was entitled to. She says that the rest of us children had more than she had.

"Well, she and my mother had breast cancer at just about the same time. They would sit around and argue about it, blaming each other for it. It was just awful. My sister would say, 'It's your fault. If I hadn't had such a miserable childhood, I wouldn't have had all this stress and this wouldn't have happened to me.' And my mother would say, 'It's all *your* fault. If you hadn't been so miserable as a kid, I wouldn't have had all that stress and this wouldn't have happened to me.' "

In Roslyn's family, conflict centered on longstanding marital issues. "My father has never treated my mother very well. But he has a cousin who treats his wife like a queen. If it was her birthday or their anniversary, the cousin would think nothing of taking her to the fanciest, most elegant restaurant in town. My father would joke about taking my mother out for a special treat—at a budget place like Howard Johnson's. He thought this was funny, but my mother never did.

"Well, a while ago the cousin's wife got breast cancer, and the cousin was just wonderful to her. He couldn't do enough for her. My mother always said how lucky she was to have a husband who treated her that way. Then, when my mother got her own cancer, my father said, 'See, you cursed yourself.' He was recalling that while the cousin's wife was sick my mother had said, 'I'd gladly give my breast to be treated like her.' "

## FACING OUR FEELINGS

Grown daughters may react pragmatically, but they also have to cope with powerful emotions, both their own and their mothers'.

"I was walking around like a zombie after I heard my mother's diagnosis," Helen says. "For several days I had no short-term memory. The hospital social worker asked me, 'Have you had a good cry yet?' I hadn't. But that seemed like an assignment, so I went home and cried. It did help me feel somewhat better. So I asked my mother, 'Have you had a good cry yet?'

"How did my mother respond to this? The way she responds to everything. She prides herself on her independence, her ability to handle things. She's proud that she's from pioneer stock. She was widowed in her early thirties and raised her kids alone. She's using that same strength now."

Helen's right. A mother reacts to cancer as she has lived her entire life. The mirror of mortal crisis reflects back her own character and beliefs, as well as her style of coping. Lee describes her mother as "stoic and proud" in the face of malignancy.

Martha calls hers "a woman of faith. We're faith people. My mother worried about her children, but she felt she would die. She accepted it and believed it was in the hands of God.

"Her faith helped us all. She taught us that whatever happens is God's will. She turned to God and said, 'Take me, I'm ready.' Whatever the doctor said, she did."

But Andrea witnessed something completely different. "My mother hasn't recovered emotionally after six years," she says. "I think she feels as though she still has cancer. She won't say the word. As soon as she was diagnosed, she seemed to assume that she was dying. She seemed at first to give up and go into mourning for herself. I encouraged her to join a cancer survivors group, but she wouldn't."

Says Jane, "My mother wouldn't talk about cancer either, to anyone outside the immediate family. She was afraid that if people knew she had it, they'd write her off. She didn't want to be written off. She went on an immediate health kick. She started really exercising and watching what she ate. She looked terrific afterward, better than she had in a long time."

Linda says, "My mother denied her mortality. She seemed to imply, 'I'll always be here.' "

These women embody the distinct styles of reaction to breast cancer that researchers at the Faith Courtauld Research Unit at King's College in London have identified.

Martha's mother's style, stoic acceptance, is probably the easiest on loving bystanders. Experts believe that relatives and friends even unwittingly encourage this outward placidity, this belief that what will be will be, rather than dealing with the jagged, jarring emotion of a woman raging against her fate.

There is no evidence that mood or attitude can affect malignant cells, but the Courtauld Unit researchers found that the stoic style in breast cancer patients is associated with relatively poorer quality of life as well as lower survival rates.[8, 9, 10] Even Martha has her doubts about how much good this did her mother. "I think that sometimes that attitude takes away from some of the human emotions you might feel. People think that showing fear, anger, and so forth shows a lack of faith."

The "hopeless-helpless" reaction of Andrea's mother is also associated with poorer outcomes. Here a woman allows her anger and depression to immobilize her rather than facing her illness as a challenge to be met. Jane's mother's fighting spirit and Linda's mother's denial are more often associated with better outcomes. The fighter confronts her illness, believing that she can affect her health; she's flexible and resourceful in this effort. The denier shows little outward distress, but neither does she try actively to cope.

The way a mother copes may not match her daughter's reactions and wishes, as Lee discovered when she tried to help her mother. "I saw a book by an artist who had had a mastectomy," Lee says. "She had made a number of photographs of herself and then beautifully embellished them, hand coloring the scar or making collages.

"I tried showing it to my mother. I wanted her to know, 'See, you're still normal. What has happened to you has not made you ugly. Here's a woman who has had the same thing happen and is proud.' But she didn't respond."

It's important for daughters to allow mothers to make sense of breast cancer in their own way. At the same time, though, the daughter can draw strength from her own appraisal of the situation.

## FACING OUR FUTURES

A diagnosis of cancer comes, as the old slogan says, on "the first day of the rest of our lives." For many daughters, it is the day the world changed—the day they learn that they belong to a high-risk group. It may be the day they begin to confront their own mortality.

"I always assumed my mother would live to eighty like her own parents did," Helen says. "Those plans played a very important part in my life. My mom lives with us and it's really worked out beautifully. Our kids are so close to her. It's almost as though we have a three-parent family.

"Her sister died of breast cancer some years ago. I don't know much about it, because she lived so far away. But now my mother has got it too.

"I always used to say to myself, 'I've got my mom until my kids are grown.' But now I wonder, do I have *myself* until my kids are grown? Having my family around me has always been very important to me. But now I'm losing my family. With my mom going, I'm losing the last of my family."

Discovering her own high-risk status has shattered Helen's sense of natural order, of family stability, of her own ability to keep her children secure.

For Marcia, whose mother died a decade ago, the loss of continuity is poignant and powerful. "As my children are growing up, I miss her more and more. The more that happens in our life as a family—the more birthdays, celebrations, holidays—the more I think she is missed. When I lost her, my children were not born. I wish they had known her. It's so important to you to have that sense."

## IN SUMMARY

We've made a number of observations about women who were adults when their mothers developed breast cancer:

- An adult daughter generally responds to her mother's illness in much more pragmatic terms than a child, who lacks the resources to respond pragmatically.

- The mother's cancer rarely becomes a central element of the daughter's identity or a developmental issue in her own life.
- Such a daughter often sees breast cancer as a feature of aging rather than of womanhood *per se*. Especially if the mother had cancer late in life, the daughter may not consider herself directly threatened until she gets much closer to her mother's age.
- The daughter's reaction often centers on providing concrete help in coping. This often takes the form of gathering information about possible treatment options.
- A woman in the early stages of adulthood, who is deeply involved in a career or her own family or both, may not be as severely affected by the early stages of her mother's cancer.
- Often a woman views her mother's possible or actual death as a break in family continuity, depriving her actual or potential children of a grandmother and her mother of grandchildren.
- Family reactions to the crisis of a mother's breast cancer occur in the context of both the mother's style of coping and the issues and personalities that mark the family.

In the final analysis, though, each daughter deals with her mother's malignancy in the only way she can: in terms of the woman she is.

"My mom kept saying, 'Don't worry about me!' " Helen remembers. "That really bothered me, because I was very upset, both for her and for myself. I thought about it a lot. And finally I said, 'I'm *going* to worry about you.' She didn't say anything, but I think that now she's accepted that I do."

# 3

❦

# *Filling Out the Family Tree*

I BELONG to a Clan of One-breasted women," states the Utah writer Terry Tempest Williams, in her recent book, *Refuge*.[1] "My mother, my grandmothers, and six aunts have all had mastectomies. Seven are dead. The two who survive have just completed rounds of chemotherapy and radiation. I've had my own problems: two biopsies for breast cancer and a small tumor between my ribs diagnosed as a 'border-line malignancy.' "

There is more to Williams's story than plain genetic bad luck. She belongs to a large Mormon family of "downwinders," living on the windward side of the sites where nuclear bombs were tested above ground in the 1950s. At the time, the government declared these areas "virtually uninhabited." The breast cancer epidemic among such "virtual uninhabitants" as Williams's kinswomen probably had its start in the brilliant man-made sunrises that lit their desert horizons and the fine, deadly dust that showered over their towns.

But Williams, who was a child when the tests were conducted, did not know about them until many years later. What she did know was that "one by one, I watched the women in my family die common, heroic deaths. We sat in waiting rooms hoping for good news, always receiving the bad. I cared for them, bathed their scarred bodies and kept their secrets. I watched beautiful women become bald, as cytoxan, cisplatin and adriamycin were injected into their veins. I held their foreheads as they vomited green-black bile and I shot them with morphine when the pain became inhuman. In the end, I witnessed their last peaceful breaths, becoming a midwife to the rebirth of their souls."

For her, "this is my family history."

## JOINING THE CLAN

What Terry Williams calls family history is a fate that does not happen to one person alone. It belongs to an entire group, and to particular members of the group precisely because they are members. It can make an individual feel herself a partner in her family's shared destiny.

If there have been multiple cancers among your close relatives, you may recognize Emily's experience. "I am the only woman in three generations of our family not to have gotten breast cancer," Emily says. "My grandmother and my aunts had it, my mother had it, and then my sister had it. When my mother had her own cancer, she was very cool, very competent, very stoical. She rarely shared her feelings about it. She just handled it.

"But my sister's cancer upset her very, very much, even more than her own, it seemed to me. She wasn't stoical. After my sister got it, she said something that shocked me very deeply. All my life I had always heard her say how much she had always wanted children, how happy she had been to have children, how much she enjoyed having children. But when my sister was sick she said to me, 'If I had known how strong this genetic trend would become in our family, I might have thought differently about having children.' "

For Emily's mother, family history is clearly a part of her identity both as a woman and as a mother. She feels a weight of inevitability, a burden of guilt over her own role as its unwitting agent.

But as we've seen in the last two chapters, and as you may know from your own experience, individuals and families react to similar situations in quite diverse ways. For many women, simply belonging to a family need not imply accepting its history as emblematic of your own. Jeannette, for example, sees her fate as quite distinct from her relatives'.

"I've outlived my mother by thirteen years and my sister by five," she says. "I don't think it's inevitable that I will get it. How do I cope with the risk? I take very good care of myself. I'm not sure they did."

The same is true for Ginnie, who sees the high incidence of cancer among her kin as a series of separate accidents, not as a pattern that dictates her own future. "I really don't feel that I'm at high risk for breast cancer, despite a mother and an aunt who died of the disease. There's been a lot of cancer in my family. But you have to look at all of it carefully. My grandfather, who died of liver cancer, worked with asbestos for forty years. My aunt, when she was a girl, had radiation treatment for acne; it was all over her shoulders. My mother had lots and lots of chest X-rays for bronchitis. My sister, who has had both thyroid and breast cancer, works with an electron microscope. I don't do any of these things. I think that environment has a lot to do with getting cancer of any kind."

Whether an individual chooses to embrace or disassociate herself from a shared family destiny or does something in between probably depends far more on her values and relationships than on her objective risk of developing breast cancer. As we'll see in Chapter 5, science can rarely predict with any certainty whom the disease will strike. Consciousness of family heritage strongly motivates many women to practice effective early detection. But finding ways to differentiate themselves from stricken relatives allows other women to distance themselves from danger. As long as they don't use this approach to justify neglecting their early detection screening, it can serve as a useful means of coping with anxiety.

Such defenses can work for a long time. But there are events that can topple them very suddenly. "At the time that my mother's mother and my mother's sister died of breast cancer," Helen says, "we had a long-distance relationship. We kept in touch on the phone. They were out West and we were here. My mother would call and my aunt would always say, 'I'm all right. Life is normal. Don't worry about me.' Up until the week she died, she was going around making life normal, trying to do everything she usually did.

"I knew about those other two breast cancers in the family, but I thought of them as something that happened to them, not something that could happen to me. As long as my mom didn't get it, she was my lineblocker. I thought, well, maybe she didn't get the genes that my aunt did. Maybe they didn't come down to me. But now, she also has been diagnosed with breast cancer. She's just finishing her course of chemo. And so I've lost my lineblocker. Now there's me."

*The second or third breast cancer in the family has, for many women, the power to transform the disease from an isolated calamity or a statistical abstraction into a direct, personal threat.* For many women, that is the time that the possibility becomes real and they begin to take action to protect themselves by starting serious programs of twice-yearly clinical breast exams, yearly mammograms, and monthly self-exams.

"When my mother died, she was fifty-three," Teresa says. "We four daughters were all in our twenties or younger. But just a few months ago, at twenty-seven, one of my sisters had something funny show up on her mammogram. This made me nervous and brought me into the breast center for surveillance."

It was the same for Martha, who is in her mid-fifties. "When my mother had her cancer some years ago, they explained about us being at high risk too. I didn't see it then as having very much to do with me directly. At that time, it was just her. She was sixty-nine years old. She was old enough to die.

"But three months ago, my sister was diagnosed with breast cancer. That scared me very much. It made the possibility seem much more real, much more connected to me. That brought me into the breast clinic for regular screening. Things have changed since my mother. For me, now, breast cancer in our family is something that's just expected. I have two other sisters. We just don't know which one of us will get it next."

Adds Abby, "I was very young when my mother had her cancer. Then my sister also developed it when I was in my twenties—she's my half sister, but we have the same mother. She's survived for eleven years now. But when she got it I really developed my fatalistic attitude."

Cindy wipes a tear as she listens. Finally she says, "My sister has had three breast cancers over almost fifteen years. But now they've found something on my mother's mammogram. She's going for her biopsy tomorrow.

"What does that say about me? It scares me. The really difficult thing is being the next to go in your particular lineup."


## ARE WE OUR SISTERS' KEEPERS?

When a woman consciously takes a place in a family "lineup," her feelings about her risk status change. But change even more drastic and pronounced often occurs when that second or third cancer in the family—or even the family's first—strikes a sister. A sibling of a woman's own sex, who shared her childhood and probably shares many of her genes, is the relative more like herself than anyone in the world.

The danger now takes on a new immediacy. It drops down to one's own generation, changing from something that happens to mothers, grandmothers, and aunts—an affliction of older women a generation removed—to something that threatens peers, contemporaries, women like oneself in one's own family, women at one's own stage of life. *Breast cancer in a sister markedly increases many women's feeling of vulnerability by making the reality of the disease plausible in their own generation.*

"My sister died of breast cancer one month ago," Chris says. "She was very courageous. She really fought it. We all thought she was going to beat it. When she didn't, I was very shaken. I always felt, you get breast cancer and you recover. That's what my experience had been up until she died. I had seen people get it and survive. But now I don't think that."

Adds Lorraine, "I've had five women friends die of breast cancer. Now my sister has it. I think, you get it and you die."

Your own experience as well as these stories may tell you that for the woman on the sidelines a sister's breast cancer has a different resonance from a mother's. Mothers model our future selves, but siblings share our lifelong present. And many sisters share, in addition, an intimacy, a level of intuitive understanding, a commonality of experience and concern that doesn't exist across generations. "I talk with my sister on the phone a lot," Cindy says. "She really needs to talk. She's living alone there with her two kids. She can't talk to them about this, and there's so much she wants to say. She can't talk with my parents either. They get so upset."

Without the constraints and issues that divide parents and children, but with the frankness of those who belong to the same generation, and the special identification of siblings, a woman often sees her sister's disease with a special clarity. And in watching the sister's reaction, many try on styles of coping to see how well they fit—just in case.

"My sister has had several different emotional reactions," Cindy says. "She has had breast cancer three times. Can you believe it? She's going through her third course of chemotherapy right now. The first time she was pretty calm, considering. She believed she would beat it. The second time she was hysterical. The third time, this time, I think she's just resigned.

"She found the first lump almost fifteen years ago. She was pretty young then—she's forty-five now. In those days, her children were small—maybe three or four, and her husband was away with his job. I don't think she did anything about the lump right away. But then her husband came home and they moved to a different state. That's when she had the first mastectomy. It was a very, very radical one. They took the muscles from her chest and under her arm.

"After that, I really think she was pretty hopeful. Then a couple of years later, she found the second lump, in the other breast. That time, it really freaked her out. And that was a terrible, really stressful time for her anyway. Just before she found the lump, her husband had told her he wanted to leave her. So here she was, with two small children, in the midst of a divorce and everything that that entailed, and facing a second mastectomy.

"It's been very hard for her. She's raised the kids by herself and had to work. But she's been wonderful—so brave and positive. And she really felt she had beaten the cancer. She's just gotten her ten-year silver plate from Reach for Recovery; she's been very involved in that.

"And then just recently, she was reading, and she looked down at her chestless chest and saw another lump. It was a terrible blow to her, a really terrible disappointment. And she's really worried about the kids. She's just finished the chemo. I just don't know how she manages."

In her epic battle against cancer, Cindy's sister has shown at various times three of the hallmark coping styles we discussed in the previous chapter, a valiant fighting spirit with touches of helplessness and stoic acceptance. But for some women in the prime middle years, denial—especially of possible death—offers a way to endure the experience.

"My sister was totally shocked by her breast cancer," Ginnie says. "When she first found the lump, she totally denied that there was going to be anything wrong with her. She went into her surgery denying that there could possibly be another cancer after she had already had thyroid cancer. So when they told her that it was malignant, and that it was bilateral, she was just totally devastated.

"She just went to pieces and couldn't do anything to cope. She was immobilized. She had to make decisions, but she just couldn't act. She's usually so well informed, so active. But this time she couldn't hold it together. I wrote to a lot of doctors to find out about the best treatments.

"Finally she started to pull herself together, to rally herself, but in a very strange way. She started insisting that the cancer wasn't entirely bad, that maybe some good would even come of it. She said it was good that she was going to have both breasts off, because she thought maybe she would have reconstruction. And she thought that when they do the reconstruction, she's going to also have them do augmentation. She says she's going to come out of this much bigger on top than she was before. She's excited about that, about being bigger.

"Her body image has always been important to her, but it's become even more important now. She's very concerned about being attractive, especially to men. She's lost her breasts, but somehow she wants to come out of this and the reconstruction with her breasts bigger and more important than ever."

Ruth has also seen denial in another, less constructive form. "My sister denies the cancer completely. She won't admit that there was anything wrong. I knew that this wasn't any good. When the women from the cancer groups came around to visit her in the hospital after her mastectomy, she refused to see them. That's when I knew that things were far worse than I had imagined. They came to see her, with their hair all done, beautifully dressed, feeling good, to help her. And she sent them all away. I said, 'Why don't you listen to them? They've gotten themselves all dressed up to come and help you.' She said, 'I don't need them.' And I said, 'Yes, but maybe they need you.'

"But she wouldn't have anything to do with them. She was pretending that she was in absolute control. She was absolutely ready to go over the edge, but she insisted on the self-delusion that she was so strong. She wasn't going to join them. She wouldn't identify with *them,* be one of the women like *them.*"

But sometimes a form of denial can lead to a form of renewal. "My sister had breast cancer a couple of years ago," Lorraine says. "Right after her operation, she had a party in her room. She invited all sorts of people, and they came to see her and partied for twelve hours. And for that whole year afterward, she felt like a queen. She looked fabulous, she felt wonderful, her husband and everyone treated her wonderfully. During that time, I was frightened for her, and it was difficult for me to deal with her. I wanted to scream and cry and get angry. It was very hard for me to deal with someone who was so up.

"But then after a year, she completely crashed. She became depressed, and the chemotherapy brought on early menopause. But she was able to pull herself together and look at her life. She thought about what was important to her. She made a lot of positive changes in her life and her relationships."

Coping mechanisms also take more drastic form. "After my sister's first mastectomy, she just kept getting lumps in the other breast," Ruth said. "It was terrible. She was always going in to have them looked at, to have them removed. There was so much stress, with finding them, and the biopsies and what have you. Finally she decided just to have all that tissue emptied out. I think it was a very wise thing to do. Why should she deal with all that stress?"

Adds Sheila, "My sister also had a prophylactic mastectomy with reconstruction. My mother had breast cancer, and they found my sister's in a very early stage. They said there were cancerous cells, but it wasn't a tumor yet. She decided to take it all off so she wouldn't have to worry about it."

Though attractive to some high-risk women, prophylactic mastectomy remains very controversial. We'll discuss it in detail in a later chapter.

## FAMILY TIES

If individuals' styles of reacting vary, so, once again, do families' styles of coping, based, as always, both on circumstances and on relationships.

"I really don't know how my sister handles the day-to-day," Cindy says. "The family's really spread out. My parents are in New England, I'm here, and she's down south. We can really only keep in touch by phone. We do a lot of phoning. I try to help her.

"And now, with my mother and my sister sick, I'm thinking more about myself. I'm divorced, and I'm really afraid that when my turn comes, I won't have any family left. I'll have to face it all alone."

For Martha, though, "our family's experience taught us how important emotional support is. Of course, we all live nearby and we're close. When my sister was going through her chemo, we would take turns going over there to spend the night with her. We would sit with her, read to her. I know that it meant a great deal to her to have us there."

And what if relationships are not warm and supportive?

"I have a strange feeling about all of this," Ginnie says. "My sister and I fought a lot as kids. You know, when you have a sister and you're fighting, there are times when you think, 'Gee, I wish I didn't have a sister.' But now when I remember that, I feel kind of guilty. I know that I certainly never wanted to be the sole surviving woman of the family.

"And there's a lot of strain with my mother. My mother and she argue all the time, so my mother wants me to tell her things. She says, 'Tell her not to have the reconstruction; the implants will give her cancer again.' Or: 'Tell her not to do this; she'll get cancer again.' Or: 'Tell her not to eat that; she'll get cancer again.' "

The same is true in Emily's family. "My sister has always been the problem person in our family. She's always been negative. She complains a lot. And when she got breast cancer, people would tell her it was because of her negative attitude. That seemed unfair and cruel to me, but it just fed into her feelings of being misunderstood.

"And her cancer has become a great concern to me in case I should get breast cancer. I know that my having the disease would be terribly, terribly painful for my mother."

And yet, Abby says, "Because of all this, I feel bonded to my sister in a weird way. The fact that we share this genetic thing bonds us. I'm sure she feels the same way. I know I could discuss all of my feelings about this with her."

## IN SUMMARY

When breast cancer strikes relatives besides one's mother, it raises a number of issues for most high-risk women:

- Multiple breast cancers in the family increase a woman's sense that the disease is inevitable.
- Breast cancer in a sister usually dramatically increases a woman's sense of vulnerability.
- A woman often identifies and closely studies a sister's coping patterns, as if trying on a style of reaction.

But in the end, it is usually simple sisterly love that prevails.

"Before she died," Chris recalls, "my sister said to the rest of us, 'You know, this could have been worse. It could have been one of you.' She said, 'It's easier to deal with having this happen to me than to someone I love. I don't think I could have handled watching it happen to one of you.'"

# II

❦

*Assessing the Risk*

# 4

❦

# *Why Do People Get Breast Cancer Anyway?*

Now it's time to move beyond the experience of cancer in the family to the task of constructing a positive response. In this section we take the first step—demystifying the nature of cancer and the concept of risk, both of which strike many people as abstract and complicated. This information, we hope, will lead you to three important conclusions: that the early detection practices we and others recommend offer the best chance of meeting the challenge of the disease, that the risk you face may be smaller than you suspect, and that your risk is to some extent under your control. Then we'll be ready, in the final section, to discuss how you can apply this knowledge in your daily life.

We start with a fact about breast cancer that tremendously increases many people's sense of vulnerability: Nobody knows what causes it. Scientists are making real progress in unraveling the processes that turn normal cells into cancerous ones, but no one has yet pinned down a definite cause. You, like many people, may have your own ideas about this question, ideas that may reflect what you've seen happen around you. Lots of the women in our sample have definite notions about why it struck their relatives. How many of these seem plausible to you?

Abby, as befits her general fatalism, ascribes the disease to "genetics and fate."

Jane takes a much less pessimistic view, blaming X-rays. "My mother's father died of TB. They were afraid she'd catch it too. When she was young, she had tons of chest X-rays. I always thought they must have contributed to her cancer. But she thought cancer had something to do with viruses. She always suspected she had caught it from a friend of hers with lung cancer that she helped take care of. Anyway, when she was sick, she didn't want to kiss her kids because she didn't want us to catch it."

For Jeannette, the crucial fact is that "my mother and sisters had a lot of stress in their lives before they got their cancers. They were all married to macho-type men who didn't allow them to grow. They kept it all inside. I try to handle stress, not to let it overwhelm me. I think that has a lot to do with staying healthy."

For Laura, the culprit is diet. "My mother grew up in Wisconsin," she recalls. "They used to eat a lot of butterfat, cream right off the top of the milk bottle, that sort of thing. She told me she read an article about how there was a high rate of breast cancer in the dairy states. She believed that the diet they used to eat contributed to her cancer."

Roslyn cites a different aspect of the foods we eat. "We don't know what chemicals there are in our food or in our environment" she worries. "All the additives and chemicals can't be any good for us."

For Ginnie, breast cancer can be an occupational hazard. "My sister's a research scientist. She's had cancers in both her neck and her breast. She uses an electron microscope all the time in her work. And she said to me just the other day, 'You know, I never thought about it before, but the microscope sheds electrons just between here' "—Ginnie's hands, one under her chin, the other below her breast, frame a crucial body area— " 'and here. Anyway, just where both my cancers were.' "

If you've been following media reports about breast cancer, you already know that every one of the factors mentioned here seems reasonable to at least some reputable researchers. But none, as far as we yet know, is the whole truth. Indeed, none of these is a "cause" in the sense that a specific microbe causes a particular infection. Current knowledge quite convincingly argues that cancer usually involves more than one causative factor because it develops through a complex, multistage process.

But the very fact that researchers are exploring so many possibilities has a downside for those concerned with preventing cancer. We're obviously still some distance from the precise understanding that would pinpoint particular causes and allow doctors to develop truly effective prevention strategies and a comprehensive cure.

And scientific uncertainty, furthermore, has an emotional effect. The experts' uncertainty feeds the uncertainty that the rest of us feel. The whole question of what causes cancer can become a Rorschach inkblot. People may see causes that reflect not only their attitude to the disease but, more broadly, to their lives in general. Some feel helpless; Abby's answer— "genetics and fate"—invokes an inevitable doom. But others see a possibility for individuals influencing their own fates. Jeannette's emphasis on styles of handling stress, Laura's on a fatty diet, place the future at least partly within human control.

You may want to examine your own attitude toward cancer. You may find that it coincides with a more general philosophic outlook you hold in life. What do you think caused your relative's cancer? Do you believe that the same factors apply to you? Do you see ways of exercising any control over the risk you face? Do you feel helpless in the face of your biochemistry or hopeful that you have a fighting chance against the disease?

A high-risk woman's attitude toward breast cancer—and toward her own life prospects generally—tends to correlate with her beliefs about breast cancer's cause, our research shows. Those who believe that they can affect the outcome of their cancer tend to see themselves in greater control of their lives generally.

## THE ENIGMA OF CANCER

Why don't we yet know the cause of cancer, when billions of dollars and decades of work have gone into the effort and when more lives could be saved if we knew? It's because the disease presents researchers with an almost unparalleled challenge, a problem as complicated as the nature of life itself. A full understanding of cancer, in fact—an explanation of why it starts and how it spreads—will require understanding the basic processes of life, the innermost mechanisms of our cells. Cancer is nothing more or less than a drastic malfunction of life's most elementary processes.

To complicate the task even further, cancer—and even breast cancer—isn't one disease, but a multitude of subtly different diseases that use the same strategy. Breast cancer, for example, occurs in about a dozen basic forms, which can combine to produce even more possibilities. Thinking of all our human cancers as a single entity, therefore, is as misleading as considering all infectious diseases—from AIDS to the common cold—as a single entity because they all involve outside invaders that use the resources of our bodies for nourishment in order to multiply.

But unlike epidemics such as smallpox and typhoid, which gave medical science its greatest successes to date, cancer uses a strategy that doesn't involve foreign attack. No alien raiders swarm through the body, ambushing our organs. No readily spotted intruders tempt the immune system's search-and-destroy apparatus. Far from being a marauding stranger, cancer is an insider, a homebody, a family member run amok.

## THE LIFE OF A TUMOR

A cancer starts when a single cell slips the controls that guide normal development. Ordinarily, our body's billions of cells are good, law-abiding citizens who follow the rules that keep things running smoothly. Each of the many types—which correspond to our many types of tissues—generally keeps to its own particular location, function, and identity. Breast cells, for example, are distinctively different from kidney or bone cells in where they're found, what they do, and how they look. When things go right, cells live cooperatively and die in their own neighborhoods.

Once in a while, though, something goes slightly haywire. Rather than the usual orderly growth, an aberrant spurt creates an abnormal clump of cells known as a tumor. But this event, neither rare nor necessarily dangerous, usually doesn't signal the start of a cancer. Most of us have harmless tumors in various spots throughout our bodies. And most of them remain localized, encapsulated—in technical terms, benign—rather "like a tangerine," in the words of one researcher.

But occasionally, a tumor begins to change, moving, in technical terms, toward the state of malignancy. Its cells abandon both their normal form and their original identities as breast or kidney or colon tissue. They change shape and size and color. Early in this process, while the growth is still technically "precancerous," pathologists can spot misshapen, oddly colored cells under the microscope. Where this can be done readily, as in the Pap smear of cervical cells, doctors can easily halt the advance toward life-threatening cancer.

But this kind of detection rarely happens with relatively inaccessible breast cells. If left to themselves the abnormal tumor cells begin to multiply aggressively, at the expense of their neighbors. They use up more than their share of nutrients. The unruly cluster expands rapidly, paying no attention to normal "turf" boundaries. At this point, with luck, a breast tumor may be large enough to appear as a tiny, anomalous spot on a mammogram.

## THE DANGER SPREADS

The ancient Greeks were the first to notice that certain types of tumors put out jagged, clawlike extensions and spread sidelong, suddenly, erratically, and unpredictably. These growths and their grasping ways reminded them of the crab, which is *karcinos* in Greek and survives in English in words such as "carcinoma" and "carcinogen." The Romans, later translating the marine metaphor into Latin, gave it their name for "crab," the word we still use, "cancer."

Just why a placid clump of cells should suddenly turn unruly is one of the deepest questions facing science today. For a combination of apparently quite complicated reasons, originally normal cells can turn into renegade cells capable of going on the attack against their normal neighbors. Cancer cells produce chemicals that give them powers unknown to ordinary breast or liver or colon cells. For a start, they can move around more freely. Then they begin to cut through surrounding tissues. Particularly aggressive cells break into the blood or lymph system and ride to distant organs, where they start new colonies, called metastases, which themselves also seed new colonies. Thus, for example, Laura's mother had cells growing in her bones that a pathologist could tell originated in her breast tumor. Teresa's mother had them in her ovaries, and Abby's sister had them in her lungs. Unchecked malignant growths eventually destroy the organs they invade and, ultimately, through metastatic spread, the person who harbors them.

Malignancies ignore all the rules of ordinary cell life. Most importantly, they do not stay in their assigned places or die at the appropriate time to make way for new cells. In these cells, many of the basic mechanisms of life itself go awry.

Although they ultimately defy the rules that govern other cells, cancers start through slight perversions of normal processes. Certain apparently normal genes present in many kinds of cells have the capacity to transform themselves into "oncogenes"—renegade genes that code for malignant rather than normal or benign growth. Why this transformation happens is now the subject of intense research. A propensity to this transformation may run in certain families. Or a mutation—a spontaneous change in a gene—may make certain originally normal genes more susceptible.

In addition, certain outside factors appear in many cases to help trigger the change of normal genes to oncogenes. Some chemicals, for example, clearly have a hand in the onset of many cancers, either by causing mutations or by helping to promote malignant growth once a mutation has occurred. Even so it's certainly not true that, as Roslyn fears, "everything causes cancer." Some types of radiation also have the power to damage genetic material and probably trigger cancerous growth. Everyone knows about cigarette smoke and lung cancer, about sunlight and skin cancer. Radioactivity also clearly increases cancer risk. But the reason that one person with a certain level of exposure develops cancer and another with an equal level does not remains buried deep within the cells.

Viruses also have special properties that can contribute to some cancers. These tiny organisms can invade our cells and insert some of their own genes into our cells' normal genetic material. Sometimes those inserted genes code for cancer and help turn a normal cell malignant. This does not mean that cancer is "catching" in the sense of an ordinary viral disease like flu or a cold, but some evidence suggests that viruses that insert their own genes may be implicated in certain malignancies. The human papilloma virus, for example, seems to push cervical cells in a cancerous direction. Venereal infections may well be implicated in certain prostate cancer as well.

However it happens, though, the shift from normal gene to oncogene still does not add up to a full-fledged cancer. The presence of normal genes that can become oncogenes merely provides the opportunity for that potentially deadly process to begin. These genes form "a keyboard on which many different carcinogens [cancer-causing agents] may play," writes J. Michael Bishop of the University of California at San Francisco Medical School, who shared the 1989 Nobel Prize in medicine for his work describing oncogenes.[1]

But why should our own cells carry genes with the potential to destroy us? Because, scientists believe, life itself depends on the characteristics of growth that cancer cells put to such harmful use. All creatures start as a single cell. In humans, as in all complex organisms, for a limited time during the embryonic stage, our cells multiply rapidly, travel freely, change identity, and found new colonies in distant places— just the things that malignancies also do with such devastating effect. But once we've stopped being embryos, the genes calling for those behaviors are supposed to shut down, probably with the aid of specially equipped neighboring genes known as suppressors. The oncogene problem may come down to a faulty "off" switch for genes that have passed their usefulness. The contributing carcinogen might either turn the oncogene back on at the wrong time or disable the suppressor that had kept the gene dormant.

## TO THE RESCUE

But just as a sperm fertilizing an egg doesn't guarantee the birth of a baby nine months later, so activating an oncogene doesn't automatically produce a cancer. For a new cancer to establish itself, several more things have to go just right—or, from the patient's viewpoint, totally wrong. The various early steps of the cancer process, in fact, appear to happen repeatedly in people who remain healthy—but most of the time, fortunately, in the wrong order or in the wrong place. Or if the cancer process does manage to get under way, the vigilant cells of the immune system spot the upstart growths and annihilate them.

Sometimes, though, the new malignancy gets some extra help. Chemical "promoters" somehow speed the process. These are chemicals that, while not themselves cancer *causing,* still encourage or assist the renegades' development. Promoters may be artificial substances like saccharin, which is related to tumor growth in animals, or substances that occur naturally in the body. Some human reproductive cancers, for example, including most breast cancers and many prostate cancers, are hormone dependent—they can't grow without infusions of the appropriate hormone, either the female estrogens or the male androgens. In hormone-dependent cancers, special receptors coat the cells' surfaces. These are special molecules designed to catch passing molecules of the appropriate sex hormone. They serve as keyholes that allow the hormone molecule, which acts like a key, to enter the cell's nucleus and nourish the malignant growth. Depriving these cells of their hormone fix by using the appropriate treatment to cut the supply or sabotage the receptors can make these cancers shrink or even disappear.

But all too often, the timing is perfect and the conditions are right. The malignancy reaches the size and stage of development that let it take its turf. It now produces chemicals that overpower or disable the cells of the immune system that ordinarily fight cancer cells. Then it can expand unimpeded.

## RACING FOR LIFE

Once this happens, the patient's fate hangs on two major factors: the stage the disease has reached when first detected, and the exact composition of the tumor. Some tumors, for example, contain more aggressive cells than others. Some tumors are made up of cells dependent on estrogen and some of cells not dependent on it.

Although there are no clean breaks in the natural history of a cancer, doctors classify malignant or cancerous breast tumors into diagnostic stages, which reflect both the size and the spread of the cancer. Staging helps determine treatment and also corresponds fairly accurately with prognosis. One commonly used staging system called TNM (an acronym for tumor, nodes, and metastases) has a four-part division. It involves examining the tumor and nodes visually and by palpation, and staging of the removed tumor and lymph nodes by a pathologist.[2] In stage I, the tumor is small, under two centimeters (about two-thirds of an inch) at its greatest extent, and the lymph nodes in the armpit, generally the first place outside the breast that the cancer spreads, contain no malignant cells. (In technical language, they are node-negative.) In stage II, the tumor is larger—two to five centimeters, about the size of a pea—and lymph nodes may or may not contain cancerous cells. By stage III, the tumor is about two inches in length or width and cancerous cells have reached the lymph nodes in the collarbone or armpit areas. There are no detectable, distant metastases. Stage III also includes tumors of any size with invasions of the skin or chest wall. By stage IV, there are obvious metastases and the tumor itself may appear as a sore on the skin or have attached itself to the chest wall. The skin surrounding the tumor has become swollen or dimpled. The lymph nodes may be positive or negative.[3]

Surgically removing an early-stage, still-localized tumor can sometimes effect a complete cure. But if cells have already begun to scatter, how many have escaped and how far they have gotten will determine whether it's possible to destroy them and stop the spread. If they've colonized far-off sites—breast cells forming a tumor in the lung, for example—they already have secondary bases for further spread. Tracking down and killing all the malignant cells may no longer be possible. The cancer has reached the stage where new tumors will grow even after the primary one is gone.

To prevent this kind of spread, in May 1988 the National Cancer Institute issued guidelines to physicians. They instructed that all breast cancer patients, even those with no known spread to the lymph nodes, should receive, along with surgery or radiation, additional therapy (technically known as adjuvant therapy) aimed at destroying cells that may have escaped.[4] Typically, this involves chemotherapy before menopause, and hormone therapy after menopause.

But experts continue to debate the wisdom of adjuvant therapy for everyone. Some 70 percent of women could survive without it and therefore don't need to endure often terrible side effects, lost work days, and expense.[5] But doctors have no way of identifying the 30 percent of women whose lives adjuvant therapy might save, a fact that convinced many experts that the benefits for the minority who need it outweigh the costs for those who don't.[5,6]

Further complicating the choice of treatment, the cells composing malignant tumors are highly variable. They not only grow wildly, they mutate wildly. A single tumor may contain cells that differ in many characteristics. Some, for example, may be extremely aggressive, others more restrained. Some may be vulnerable to certain anticancer drugs, others much less so. And as a tumor grows, internal diversity grows. Early in its life, shortly after it begins to grow, it consists mainly of young, rapidly proliferating cells. With passing time, the early members age, and older, more slowly proliferating cells account for an ever larger proportion of the total tumor mass. But anticancer drugs work best against cells growing so quickly that they hungrily gobble up any available nourishment. So the drugs take their biggest toll against newer, smaller tumors that have many young, actively proliferating cells.

An early start to treatment, therefore, obviously gives patients their best shot at a cure. With breast cancer, finding a tumor in the localized stage rather than that of distant spread more than quintuples a woman's chances of surviving five years after diagnosis. Ninety-one percent of women diagnosed with stage I breast tumors are alive five years later according to the Cancer Statistics Branch of the National Cancer Institute; 69 percent of those diagnosed at stages II and III, and 19 percent of those diagnosed at stage IV survive five years after diagnosis.[7]

But even with modern screening and detection devices, most cancers—including many breast cancers—show up only after some spread has begun. Data from the National Health Interview Survey, a continuing household survey conducted by the National Center for Health Statistics, tell us that many women—including far too many high-risk women—simply fail to have regular mammograms and clinical breast exams or to practice self-examination. Poor women in particular often receive less than adequate preventive care, a lack that shows up in a death rate from breast cancer that is 25 percent higher than that of their nonpoor counterparts. At diagnosis, they are less likely to have localized cancers, and five years later they have a poorer survival rate. Black women, in addition, suffer higher breast cancer mortality than whites. White women get the disease 20 percent more often than blacks, but black women have significantly worse chances of survival (68 percent as opposed to white women's 78 percent) and a lower chance of having localized disease (41 percent to white women's 49 percent).[8] Despite these conspicuous failures, however, today's detection techniques, though still not perfect, can vastly improve our chances of finding cancers in the early, readily curable stages.

The particular nature of her cancer also affects a patient's chances of survival. If it is very aggressive, she faces much worse prospects than she would if it were slower spreading—and she will need much more aggressive treatment if she is to have a chance at survival.

The presence or absence of estrogen receptors on the cells also relates to long-term chances. Approximately two-thirds of breast cancer patients have cancer cells coated with special molecules that can catch passing hormone molecules. These receptors indicate that their cancer cells need estrogen to grow, and because of that these women have a better outlook for survival than the third of breast cancer patients who lack receptors. Therapies that manipulate hormone levels help about half of all those with estrogen-dependent cancers. Premenopausal women more often lack estrogen receptors than older and postmenopausal ones; this may partially explain why cancers in young women often appear particularly virulent. Black women between thirty and forty-four have an even higher rate of estrogen receptor negative breast cancers than do whites which may partially account for the disparity in survival rates.[9] This certainly underlines the importance of all women practicing effective early detection.

## ON THE ATTACK

Scientists, as Pogo the comic-strip possum used to say, "have met the enemy and it is us." The most diabolical obstacle to destroying cancer cells is that they are *our* cells. Almost everything that kills them also kills normal cells. And that is why many cancer treatments carry such terrible side effects. To destroy abnormal cells so much like our normal ones, doctors must use chemicals that literally make the patients sick. Today, in addition to surgical removal of cancer cells, doctors depend on two standard forms of treatment: chemotherapy, poisoning tumors with chemicals; and radiotherapy, blasting them with X-rays or radioactivity. For those breast cancers that thrive on estrogen, manipulating hormone levels can also help without causing toxic side effects.

The first promising anticancer chemical, nitrogen mustard, was a potent poison that turned up during World War II poison-gas research. To this day, useful therapies still carry a toll of hideous toxicity—overpowering nausea, pain, hair loss, extreme malaise, weakness, and fatigue.

Still, scientists continue the search for poisons marginally more deadly to cancer cells than to normal ones. The key word is "marginally"; the art of chemotherapy lies in finding compounds that will kill the cancer but not the patient. The most effective dose is the very largest the patient can stand physiologically. This may be larger than the patient's ability or willingness to tolerate the side effects. Many doctors, in fact, give lower than the theoretically optimal doses because patients simply can't stand them.

But because large doses improve survival, research attention has lately turned to finding techniques that protect patients from the worst ravages of high-powered drugs. Removing some of a woman's bone marrow—a vital tissue often killed by anticancer chemicals—then replacing it after chemo, along with agents to encourage it to multiply, has proved successful in certain experimental cases. The woman could then take ordinarily fatal doses of drugs against the cancer, but survive the experience thanks to her freshly replenished supply of marrow.

## IMPROVING CHANCES OF SURVIVING

Have overall survival rates climbed in recent years? Experts disagree, some saying they have and others saying that apparent improvements are statistical flukes. There's no disagreement, though, that detection techniques are better than even a few years ago and that if women would take advantage of them, more lives could be saved. The Health Insurance Plan Study, for example, which followed 62,000 New York women starting in 1962, proved the benefits of routine screening for breast cancer, particularly of combining mammograms and clinical breast exams. A third of the breast cancers would not have been found without mammography; 45 percent would not have been found without physical exams. The study also proved that a regular program of screening finds cancers earlier. Fifty-seven percent of the cancers in women who got regular screening were found before the nodes became involved, but only 45 percent of those in the women who didn't get screened regularly. And screening turned up fully 71 percent of the cancers. Eighteen years on, the study found that screening had reduced mortality by 25 percent in women

both above and below age fifty. Regular early detection practices, therefore, clearly save lives, regardless of a woman's
age.[10,11]

It is just as clear that today's standard techniques have
saved or extended millions of lives. Almost 75 percent of breast
cancer patients now survive at least five years after diagnosis,
an encouraging advance over 1960 when approximately 60
percent survived five years. But because science still doesn't
understand the root cause of breast cancer, no available treatment corrects the conditions that cause the disease in the first
place. Surgical, chemical, and radiological search-and-destroy
are inherently stopgap measures, but for now they are the best
that doctors have to offer.

The next decade or so looks exceptionally promising. In
the past decade, biological knowledge of cells and how they
work has exploded. Researchers are now poised to exploit
their new insights and hope that someday soon they can un-
tangle the chain of events leading to cancer. And when that
happens, doctors will finally be able to attack cancer at its
sources, as antibiotics do with bacterial diseases. Treatments
will go far beyond today's methods to exploit the very structure and function of our cells themselves. Scientists hope to
marshal the body's own immune defenses—which they hope
also to strengthen through various clever techniques—to van-
quish the marauders and possibly even to reach into the chro-
mosomes to flip the right chemical switches to turn the whole
process off. They also hope to distinguish with much more
accuracy who is at risk for what type of tumor.

One promising attempt at preventing cancer begins in
1992, as the NCI undertakes a clinical trial testing whether
long-term treatment with tamoxifen, a synthetic compound
that blocks the action of estrogen on breast cells, can reduce
the rate of breast cancer in high-risk women. So far, the drug
has worked effectively as an adjuvant therapy in women with

cancers confined to the breast and axillary (armpit) lymph nodes.[12] The trial, run by the National Surgical Adjuvant Breast and Bowel Project, a research collaborative group that studies breast and colon cancer, will also test whether tamoxifen has the additional benefits of reducing the death rate from breast cancer and lowering the rates of heart attacks and bone fractures, two major causes of illness and death in women over sixty.

Sixteen thousand women who face elevated risk for breast cancer will take either tamoxifen or a placebo daily for five years. Although tamoxifen has proved effective both in extending the lives of women with breast cancer and in preventing the growth of new cancers, its side effects—nausea, hot flashes, swelling, depression, and vaginal irritation—make it a controversial treatment for healthy persons. Although 95 percent of women appear to tolerate it well, the depression has caused some to drop out of previous trials of the drug.[12] In addition, critics have questioned the wisdom of exposing healthy people over long periods to a drug that may increase the risk of other cancers.

In June 1991, the Congressional Caucus for Women's Issues challenged the National Cancer Institute and the medical research community to meet five goals by the year 2000: (1) to understand the cause and find a cure for breast cancer; (2) to lower the incidence rate significantly; (3) to cut the mortality rate by 50 percent; (4) to ensure that all woman over forty have regular mammograms; and (5) to ensure that all mammograms meet the highest standards of accuracy.[13]

These goals are not unreasonable. By the turn of the century, we may face significantly less danger from breast cancer. For now, women at risk are left with hope and a disconcertingly long list of possible culprits. Every suggested cause we heard at the beginning of the chapter is a suspect, but none has been convicted of causing cancer beyond a reasonable doubt.

Most sisters and daughters of breast cancer patients, and most women who eat butter, take chest X-rays, live stressful lives, and eat artificial preservatives will never experience the lump that can threaten their lives. They may worry about breast cancer as long as they live, but the majority of them will die of other causes.

## IN SUMMARY

The facts about cancer that a high-risk woman needs to remember are these:

- The cause of breast cancer is not yet known.
- A cancer originates in a particular body organ, such as the breast, and then spreads to other organs by a process known as metastasis. If left unchecked, this process will eventually kill the patient.
- Cancers that have not spread are much more easily and successfully treated than those that have metastasized.
- For breast cancers that have not yet spread, long-term survival rates top 90 percent. After spread has begun, however, the chances of survival are much lower.
- Early diagnosis, before metastasis has begun, gives the best chance of survival. Early detection procedures, therefore, provide the best insurance of continued breast health.

# 5

❦

# *What Is Risk?*

ABBY AND Jeannette have a lot in common. Each has lost her mother to breast cancer. Each has also had a sister get the disease (Abby 's survived, Jeannette's did not). Each knows she faces an elevated risk for the disease. But from there out they starkly disagree.

Jeannette doesn't believe she'll get it. "In 1983 my husband died suddenly of a heart attack. Three months later my sister got breast cancer. A few months later my son was in a car accident and very ill. He was totally paralyzed for a while. He eventually got better, but the stress was terrible. I think if I didn't get cancer during that year, I'm not going to."

Abby is just as convinced that she will. "Usually I think that since my mother and sister both got it, I will too. Sometimes I wonder whether so many other people getting it might protect me—by a kind of law of averages. But basically I feel that it's inevitable, only a matter of time."

Who's right? Who has the better grasp on the reality of risk? Who has the more accurate assessment that will maximize both her ability to take reasonable precautions and her peace of mind?

The fact is: neither one. Jeannette errs in one direction,

Abby in the other, and both ignore important aspects of their own situation.

A more accurate assessment would help them both. No one is simply "at elevated risk for breast cancer." Different individuals face different degrees of danger, based on the specifics of their own lives and family trees. And no one's risk remains level over an entire lifetime. Knowing the facts might shake Jeannette's assurance a bit, but it could also help rescue Abby from her corrosive despair.

Jeannette and Abby both base their estimates on the tiny samples that their own lives provide. But epidemiologists—scientists who study the factors that influence the frequency of disease—have created mathematical models based on thousands of cases and decades of experience. They can now state much more precisely the degree of risk a given person may face. No one, of course, can name who will ultimately fall ill. But studying probabilities derived from large samples allows us to ground our thinking in something far more solid than hope or fear.

Complacent Jeannette and pessimistic Abby both misjudge their true chances. Jeannette, in her early sixties, underestimates the reality that *risk of breast cancer rises with age, especially after age sixty or sixty-five.* Despite her apparent good luck in 1983, she needs to increase, not lessen, her vigilance in practicing early detection. Abby, deeply affected by her family's suffering, ignores the fact that *the odds of not getting breast cancer are almost always much better than the odds of getting it, even for very high-risk women.* Even though each individual accumulates risks during her lifetime and the incidence of breast cancer in the general population also continues to rise, we must remember that most women, and even most high-risk women, never develop breast cancer at all. "The observed risk has rarely exceeded 30 percent in any study," concludes a team of experts at the National Cancer Institute.[1] Despite Abby's family's terrible experience, she need not live as if under an irrevocable sentence.

Estimates of breast cancer risk have become increasingly refined in recent years. But still, for all the apparent precision of the charts and numbers, for all their impressive decimal points and percentage signs, there's no such thing as certainty in any discussion of this disease. The basic causes remain unknown, although scientists now have some strong hunches.

These hunches are based on epidemiological studies clearly showing that people with certain characteristics are more likely to get the disease than people who lack these characteristics. Such characteristics are called risk factors. Risk factors, however, are not the same thing as causes. They do not necessarily cause or give you the disease; rather, they indicate a statistical relationship between a characteristic and a higher incidence of the disease. For example, as we saw in the last chapter, black women are at higher risk of dying of breast cancer than white women (though at lower risk of getting the disease in the first place). But it's not a specifically racial factor that makes black women's cancer more frequently fatal. Rather, poor women who receive inadequate preventive health care and are diagnosed at later stages of the disease face higher likelihoods of dying of cancer than prosperous women. Because a larger proportion of black than white women have low incomes, more of them get substandard care.[2,3]

By studying very large groups—thousands or tens of thousands—scientists can discover if there are traits more common among people who have a particular disease than among people who do not. Just this type of study, for example, revealed that people who get breast cancer are more likely to have relatives with the disease than are people who don't have breast cancer. The individuals who have any risk factor obviously have a greater chance of getting the condition associated with it. Large group studies also permit scientists to see how much greater that chance is. Among similarly sized groups with and without the risk factor, does the high-risk group get it twice as often? Ten times as often? A hundred times as often? How many times, in other words, does the risk factor raise a person's risk?

We've often heard (and quoted) the American Cancer Society's statistic, presented in *Cancer Facts and Figures—1991,* that one American woman in nine will get breast cancer; or, put another way, that the average woman has a one in nine chance. That doesn't mean, however, that someone whose family history doubles or triples her risk has three chances in nine or one chance in three on that basis alone. For now, it's important just to remember that the one in nine figure does not provide an accurate basis for computing any individual's chances. We'll explain why after we've given you some information that you need to understand first.

## RISK FACTORS

We're going to start off by specifying exactly what are the risk factors that science has found to be associated with a higher chance of getting breast cancer. Here are the major ones:

• Gender—More than 99 percent of breast cancers occur in women (but some do occur in men).
• Age—The longer a woman lives, the likelier she is to get breast cancer. But even so, it is the number one cause of death in women between thirty and fifty and the number two cause, after cardiovascular disease, for women over fifty, according to the National Center for Health Statistics.[4]
• Personal history of breast cancer—Women who have had breast cancer in the past have a higher than average risk of getting it again. Cancer in a single breast quintuples the risk of

a future cancer. For these women, risk rises if the original cancer occurred before age fifty, if other relatives have had premenopausal cancer in both breasts, or if a breast biopsy shows precancerous tissue.[5]

• Family history—A mother or sister who has had breast cancer doubles or triples a woman's risk. If that cancer was premenopausal or affected both breasts, the risk rises higher.[6,7] Dr. Patricia T. Kelly, a medical geneticist who has developed a procedure for analyzing breast cancer risk, has found that women who have two sisters with bilateral premenopausal breast cancer face a 50 percent lifetime risk, while the risk drops seven percentage points for women with two sisters who had postmenopausal cancer in one breast.[8]

• Hormonal factors

Age at first menstruation—Women who first menstruate at fourteen or older have 20 percent less chance of developing breast cancer than those who first menstruated before twelve.[9]

Childbearing—Women who bear a child have less risk than those who do not.[8]

Age at first childbirth—Women who give birth before eighteen have one-fourth less chance of getting breast cancer than women who do not have a child until near thirty. Those who first give birth after thirty have a greater risk than those who never give birth at all.[5]

Age at menopause—Late menopause (after age fifty) doubles a woman's risk. Surgical menopause (removal of the ovaries) before age forty-five appears to reduce risk.[9]

Except for age at childbirth and surgical menopause, there is nothing we can do about these factors. And the chance to influence our statistical risk of breast cancer would rarely weigh very heavily in such big decisions as having either a baby or major surgery. But evidence strongly suggests that factors we can much more easily influence—lifestyle choices we make every day, such as diet and exercise—may also affect our likelihood of breast cancer.

## FINDING RISKS

The first risk factor for breast cancer ever identified may strike you as odd. Around 1700, the Italian physician Bernardino Ramazzini noticed that members of religious orders got the disease more often than other women. "Tumors of this sort," he wrote in a book now recognized as the pioneering study of lifestyle's effects on health, "are found in nuns more often than in any other women. Every city in Italy has several religious communities of nuns, and you seldom can find a convent that does not harbor this accursed pest, cancer, within its walls."[10]

And why this special susceptibility? "These [tumors] are not caused by suppression of the menses [a common theory at the time], but by their celibate life," Ramazzini theorized in an observation that, slightly modified, still stands. "I have known several cases of nuns who came to a pitiable end from terrible cancers of the breast," he went on; in his time, no cancer patient ever survived.

Ramazzini may have written of nuns, but he had isolated the same underlying factor as modern-day epidemiologists who write about age at menarche, first birth, and menopause. All these factors tap into a single physiological fact: estrogens fuel most breast cancers. A woman's degree of exposure to the hormone seems related to her level of risk.

But what determines estrogen exposure? One important factor, obviously, is the amount of time it circulates at high levels in her system, which is another way of saying the number of menstrual cycles she undergoes. This era begins with menarche, ends with menopause, and is interrupted by each pregnancy. So those milestones of womanhood serve, to some extent, as benchmarks of risk. The length of the interval between menarche and first birth also seems significant to breast health. For reasons not yet clear, a short interval appears to decrease risk and a long one to increase it. Perhaps our grandmothers and great-grandmothers had a lower incidence of breast cancer than we do because their lives matched today's hormonal criteria for lower risk: first period in mid-teens, marriage in late teens, first baby within the year.

But we late-twentieth-century women are better fed, better educated, and proud of our broader opportunities. Today's well-nourished middle-class girl menstruates years earlier than she would have a century ago. Today's ambitious young woman might marry a decade and a half after her first period and give birth for the first time years after that. Does our new timetable contribute to our own rising incidence of breast cancer, which is especially sharp among the educated?

In Ramazzini's time, nearly everyone menstruated late and gave birth early and often. The few exceptions lived mainly in convents. The effect he observed derived not from celibacy, as he thought, but from childlessness (although in his time, the former was the only reliable method of achieving the latter). Ramazzini could not, however, have observed another modern trend that results in an even higher risk—and that may eventually boost breast cancer incidence rates even higher than they are today. In Ramazzini's time, a first baby in the thirties or later—an age when most women were becoming grandmothers—probably happened too rarely to figure in anyone's statistics. Today, however, as more and more women start families after thirty, a scientific consensus is growing that this trend raises risk more than never conceiving at all.

In Ramazzini's time, and, indeed, in our grandmothers',

only nature's cycles determined the dose of estrogen a woman received. In our time, estrogen also comes from the drugstore, both as birth control pills and postmenopausal replacement therapy. What does modern tinkering with the endocrines do to breast cancer risk? After decades of statistical studies, researchers are still not sure. Many years of study of oral contraceptives have produced no firm conclusion. Some experts believe that using the Pill before giving birth to a child and long-term use of oral contraceptives sharply increase risk, as do family history and benign breast disease. These scientists point out that tumors usually take more than fifteen years after contact with the carcinogen to appear at all, and that incidence doesn't top out until three decades later. The first generation of American Pill takers is just entering that peak period. But other researchers argue that given the millions of women involved, any major effect would have been obvious by now.[11,12,13] Hormone replacement therapy after menopause may well carry some increased breast cancer risk, especially after extended use. The connection between postmenopausal estrogens and endometrial cancer is well established.[1,14,15]

In 1989, a team at the National Cancer Institute headed by Dr. Mitchell H. Gail and associates developed a mathematical model of breast cancer risk and did not include either the Pill or hormone replacement therapy.[16] But that does not mean that these treatments definitely carry no risk, only that if they do, epidemiologists don't yet agree on how to measure it.

Family history is another broad category that may tap into a number of factors. We've already discussed genetic mechanisms in detail in the last chapter. But genes may also contribute to cancer only indirectly. For example, they at least partly determine when our periods begin and when they end. But other family factors may also be at work. The way to cancer may be through the stomach, not the genome. It's not known whether this represents a genetic predisposition, a lifestyle factor such as diet, or some other unknown factor. Food habits tend to span generations; the style of eating we learned at the family table, and probably share with our mothers and sisters, may be to blame.

This reminds us of Laura's mother, who blamed her cancer on the rich dairy diet of her Midwestern girlhood. International comparison studies clearly bear out her suspicions. Countries where people eat a lot of fat, such as the United States and nations of northern Europe, have much higher breast cancer rates than countries where they eat less, such as those in the Far East.[17] When we compare Americans, whose diets consist of 40 percent fat, with the Japanese, who consume one-third that amount, we find that the incidence of breast cancer in Japanese women is proportionately smaller.[18] Fat, as we've seen, plays an important role in the economy of femaleness; it appears to play a role in reproductive cancers too—including prostate cancer. And overweight women face a higher breast cancer risk than slender ones.[19,20,21] Once again, science so far provides us only an association, not a mechanism of carcinogenesis. Some scientists suspect a still-unknown connection between fat, both in the diet and on the body, and the level of circulating sex hormones.[22,23]

But Oriental diets differ from American diets in other ways than being leaner. One difference that currently interests researchers is the large quantities of cruciferous vegetables—cabbage, broccoli, cauliflower, bok choy, and others—that Far Eastern diets contain. These vegetables contain a compound that helps deactivate estrogen by breaking it down to a form unable to fuel tumors.

But is this the connection? Can we protect ourselves by simply cutting down on fats and boosting the broccoli? Not necessarily, though it certainly can't hurt. However, changing eating habits in adulthood may not do the trick, as studies of countries where incidence has risen gradually throughout this century would suggest. Year of birth strongly influences risk in these results, implying that the carcinogenic influences began very early in life, perhaps even before birth. This may indicate a strong influence of home environment, probably including diet. And since mothers, daughters, and sisters share a home for many years, it may also suggest that family tendency is more than genetic. So changing our families' diets now may not help our generation, but it might help our daughters and granddaughters.

Scientists not only study fat. They also study lean. And they draw conclusions about the effects of fat by observing the effects of its absence. Rose Frisch and her colleagues at the Harvard Center for Population Studies in 1985 found that college athletes have less breast cancer in later life than classmates who sat on the sidelines.[24] Those who exercise regularly after they graduate appear to run a lower risk. By exercise, researchers mean not the occasional game of tennis or golf, but regular aerobic training sessions at least three times a week. The reason, once again, shows the apparent connection between estrogen balance and body fat—the leaner the body, the lower the level of circulating estrogens.

What we drink may affect our cancer risk even more than what we eat. A number of studies show that alcohol is not good for breast health and that the damage relates almost directly to the number of drams consumed. At Harvard School of Public Health, Dr. W. Willett and colleagues studied the eating and drinking habits of nearly 90,000 nurses.[25] Among women with no other risk factors, even moderate drinking—three to nine glasses of wine, beer, or whiskey a week—increased risk by about 30 percent; more than nine drinks, by about 60 percent. No increase in risk was detected in women consuming fewer than three drinks per week. For high-risk women, though, alcohol consumption did not increase already elevated levels of risk. But among low-risk women under fifty-five who had more than nine drinks every week, the effect was even more drastic, more than doubling their risk compared to low-risk teetotalers of their own age.[26] A 1987 follow-up study of the first National Health and Nutrition Examination Survey found that a drinker's age affected her risk.[27] Drinking raised a woman's risk by 50 percent as compared to a similar woman who didn't drink, but the association between alcohol consumption and breast cancer was stronger for younger, premenopausal women. As the lack of uniformity in these results makes clear, scientists still do not completely understand the relationship between alcohol and breast cancer. But high-risk women can draw two conclusions from these studies. First, drinking doesn't improve breast cancer risk. Second, young women face the greatest potential harm. Wisdom would therefore counsel moderation in drinking.

Benign breast disease may be the most controversial factor so far. While some authorities imply that fibrocystic disease increases cancer risk, others disagree.[28] But exactly who has fibrocystic disease remains controversial. Some people use the term to include all women whose breasts feel lumpy at various times during the month, a category that includes half of all women of childbearing age.[29] Others restrict it to women with specific noncancerous conditions such as cysts, benign tumors, and intraductal papillomas.

Cysts, which are sacs full of fluid, may be too small to be seen without the microscope or large enough to feel with the hand. When touched they move and feel round and soft. Benign tumors, which are called either fibroadenomas or adenofibromas, also move and feel rubbery. Women between twenty and forty are likeliest to have them, and black women twice as likely as white.[30] Intraductal papillomas, which resemble warts and grow in the breast ducts, often cause bleed-

ing from the nipple. They generally occur between the ages of
forty-five and fifty, near the nipple.[31] Researchers have not yet
established a clear relationship between these conditions and
later breast cancer.[28,32] Nor have scientists established a relationship between caffeine reduction, vitamin E intake, and
reduction of breast pain, swelling, or lumpiness. Dr. Susan
Love in her *Breast Book* reviews the caffeine and vitamin E
research, pointing out that there is little scientific basis for the
commonly held idea that reducing caffeine or increasing vitamin E reduces benign breast symptoms. Nonetheless, many
women continue to report benefits from these practices.[33]

Atypical hyperplasia, a relatively rare and much more serious precancerous condition, may account for the bulk of the
risk attributed to benign breast disease, according to a 1985
Vanderbilt University study of some 10,000 biopsies. Having
a mother, sister, or daughter with breast cancer as well as
atypical hyperplasia produced a ninefold increase in risk. Still,
report the researchers, over twenty-five years, only 40 percent
of the extremely high-risk women who had both these factors
ever developed breast cancer, and two-thirds of those survived
the disease.[34]

What of Jane's idea that her mother's breast cancer came
from childhood chest X-rays? Statistics once again support her
suspicions. Along with bone marrow and the thyroid, breast
tissue is among the most sensitive to radiation, especially in
young women; here again we see youth's ability to magnify a
carcinogen's power. And radiation risk appears to mount with
the amount of youthful exposure. But does that mean that
routine mammography poses a danger? Two facts argue
against that possibility. First, modern equipment emits very
low doses of X-rays. Second, older tissues seem less affected.
For women over forty, any carcinogenic effect of mammography seems negligible.[1]

## DOING THE NUMBERS

Now that we know what the risk factors are, it's time to explore what risk itself is. In scientific usage, it's nothing more than a statistical association between a particular characteristic and a given outcome. It is a means of comparing how often a given condition occurs in different groups of people. Ramazzini observed, for example, that religious women got breast cancer more often than married ones. But even so, most nuns did not develop tumors, and some wives did. (It's important to keep in mind that calculations of risk statements always reflect incidence within a particular group; how often does breast cancer happen, for example, among one thousand nuns as opposed to one thousand married women?) A risk statement cannot select the individuals who will be affected. It is not a guarantee any more concrete than the weather forecast, which is also based on a system of comparing the known associations between various atmospheric conditions and various kinds of weather. Although it can indicate the level of risk faced by persons like you, it certainly can't tell whether you personally will be affected.

Nor do risk data tell us *why* something happens, only *what* has happened in the past. They identify an association, not a cause—an important distinction to remember as we proceed. To illustrate how the notion of risk works, let's continue discussing the weather.

Let's suppose, for the sake of this example, that you live in a dry part of the country where it rains twenty days a year. And let's further suppose that rainfall is distributed evenly throughout the year. Thus, the incidence of rainy days is 20 out of 365, and on any given day your town's absolute risk is slightly under 5.5 percent. (Absolute risk is just another way of expressing the rate of incidence.)

Now let's suppose that you have a friend who lives in a very wet part of the country, where it rains 60 days a year. The incidence of rainy days in her town is 60 in 365 or about 16.5 percent. As these numbers indicate, in any given year, your friend is three times as likely to hoist her umbrella as you are. In the jargon of epidemiology, her town's *relative risk* of rainy days is three times yours, or 3.0 as compared to yours. Relative risk is a comparison between two incidence rates.

Now let's assume that the average number of rainy days for the nation at large is 40. The average incidence of rainy days, therefore, is 40 in 365, or just under 11 percent. Even though there may be no actual town in the country that experiences exactly 40 days of rain every year, if you take the average for all the towns in the country, it comes out to 40.

Up to now we have only compared your town and your friend's town. But we can also compare either or both to the average as well, which will give us a somewhat different bit of information. Your friend's very wet hometown, for example, may have a relative risk of rain of 3.0 as compared to yours, but compared to the national average, it has a relative risk of rain of only 1.5; that is to say, the wet town has 50 percent more rainy days than the national average. Your town, on the other hand, has a relative risk of rainy days that is 0.33 as compared to your friend's town; you are one-third as likely as your friend to experience rain. But compared to the national average, your town has a relative risk of rain of 0.5; you are half as likely to experience a rainy day as the average town. A town with an incidence of rain exactly like the national average would have a relative risk of 1.0.

If you have followed this example, you understand the basic concepts of relative risk. You may want to go back over it before proceeding, because these ideas will make all the numbers you will hear about breast cancer come clear. The basic point is this: *Relative risk is a comparison of the incidence of an event within a particular group with some standard, either another group or the average for the general population.* In reading risk statistics, be sure to notice what comparisons are being made.

Epidemiologists apply these same concepts to the incidence of disease, including breast cancer. Through studying backgrounds of women who get breast cancer, they have assigned numerical values to risk factors such as age at menarche or family history of breast cancer. Please keep in mind also that our weather example does not include multiple risk factors. In a scientific discussion of a disease like breast cancer, however, multiple risk factors come into play and sometimes interact in unpredictable ways, as we saw particularly strikingly in the alcohol studies.

Please also remember that in our weather example we used the number twenty to represent the minimum or "background" incidence of rainfall. We did not discuss a locale where it simply never rains. In discussions of diseases such as breast cancer, risk determinations also take into account a minimum or background incidence, which may either be the rate of occurrence in the general population or the population composed of persons with no known risk factors. About 70 percent of breast cancers, in fact, occur in women who have no known risk factors.

Thus, risk statements about women with known risk factors assign numerical values to those risks based on the experience of large groups of persons. To illustrate, we will use risk estimates developed in a study by Dr. Mitchell H. Gail and associates at the National Cancer Institute.[16] In that study, the researchers found that the number of a woman's first-degree relatives (mother, sisters, and daughters) who have had breast cancer, her age at onset of menstruation, her age at first birth, and number of breast biopsies strongly influence her relative risk. If we consider Cindy, Abby, and Ruth, for example, we can see the effect of relatives. Abby and Cindy have both a mother and a sister who have had breast cancer, but Ruth has only a sister with the disease. (In the NCI figures, age at first birth interacts with number of relatives with cancer to affect relative risk. Abby and Cindy are comparable in this regard because both had a first child between the ages of twenty-five and twenty-nine.) With one family member who has had breast cancer, Ruth's relative risk for these two interacting factors is 2.75; Cindy's and Abby's, with two family members, is 4.9. Thus, Ruth is between twice and three times as likely as a woman in the general population to develop breast cancer and a bit more than half as likely as Cindy and Abby. Cindy and Abby are about five times as likely as a woman in the general population and a bit less than twice as likely as Ruth.

If we consider another risk factor, age at menarche, we see that Cindy, who started her periods at the late age of fourteen, has for this factor a relative risk of 1, or equal to the general population's. Ruth, who started at the age of eleven, has for this factor a relative risk of 1.2, or about 20 percent higher than the general population's. For the three factors that we have been discussing, we can place Ruth's total relative risk at approximately 3.3 (the product of multiplying 1.2 times 2.75) and Cindy's and Abby's at 4.9 (the product of multiplying 4.9 times 1.0) as compared to the general population's.

These figures may sound alarmingly high, especially Abby's and Cindy's. To find out what they really mean, we will now review the average risk that a forty-year-old American woman will face this year. What do you suppose it is? According to a 1990 study by Dr. P. C. Stomper and colleagues, it's only one in 1,200. That means that in a group of 1,200 women selected randomly for risk factors, there would be one breast cancer this year.[35] As women age, their risk increases. A fifty-year-old has a one in 600 risk of developing breast cancer, while a sixty-year-old's risk decreases to one in 400.

Thus, when we say that Ruth's family history and menstrual history approximately triple her risk or give her a relative risk of 3.30 as compared to the low-risk woman, what do we mean? Do we mean that she faces about three times the risk of the average woman, or three in 1,200? We do not, because *the average already includes all the high-risk women*. No, we mean that she faces three times the risk of the woman who does not have this risk factor, or three in 1,500, or one chance in 500. (This is certainly still a chance worth guarding against, because someone will get breast cancer. We just can't say who.)

By now it should be clear, however, that risk is a concept far more abstract than many people believe. It's important to understand, in addition, that the numbers assigned in risk assessment studies are less precise than they appear because science does not fully understand all the factors involved in breast cancer. Risk assessments cannot predict anyone's future. They can only indicate situations where caution is advisable.

## THE NUMBERS GAME

Frustratingly for Jeannette, Abby, Cindy, Ruth, and every other woman concerned about her future, discussions of risk have a slippery feel. They involve probabilities, not predictions; comparative values, not known quantities; surmises, not certainties.

Up to now we have been discussing a woman's chance of getting cancer this year, and you've probably found that chance remarkably small. So whence comes that oft-cited figure of one woman in nine provided by the *Cancer Facts and Figures—1991* volume of the American Cancer Society?[36] Because every woman's chances increase with age, and because every woman's lifetime chance is the total of all her yearly chances, the lifetime chance is obviously larger than any single year's. This one in nine lifetime figure, in fact, is the sum of the mythical average woman's chances. To be precise, it represents the mythical average woman's statistical average chances calculated over the longest possible lifetime, 110 years.

But who makes these calculations? The risk figures that we have been using in this chapter, developed by Dr. Gail and associates, are based on the Breast Cancer Detection Demonstration Project, which studied 285,000 women.[37] The team used risk factors of age at menarche, age at first live birth, number of previous breast biopsies, and number of first-degree relatives with breast cancer to estimate a woman's chance of developing breast cancer at a given age.

According to the NCI model, Abby, whose various risk factors, including menstrual and birth history and number of benign biopsies, produce a relative risk of just over 8.0 at her present age of forty, has about a 10 percent probability of breast cancer in the next decade. A forty-year-old with a relative risk of 1.0—in the NCI study, a risk equal to the average for the population—has a probability of only 1.2 percent for the next decade. (At age twenty, Abby's ten-year probability was only one-half of one percent and her low-risk counterpart's too small to measure. At fifty, Abby's ten-year probability will be about 14 percent and her thirty-year probability about 35 percent.) Statistically at least, Abby has a very good chance of avoiding breast cancer altogether. Her low-risk age mate, assuming she develops no additional risk factors over a long lifetime, will fare even better. She enters her fifties with a 1.6 percent ten-year probability and a 4.4 percent thirty-year probability.

But as anyone who has lived in the real world knows, very few people's lives go perfectly, so many people probably face a relative risk of more than 1.0. And the interaction of risk factors, as we have seen, can be very complex indeed. A number of researchers are working on further refining today's predictive models. In addition to the NCI group, Dr. Patricia T. Kelly of the San Francisco Children's Hospital has developed a system for analyzing the risk faced by relatives of cancer patients.[38] Since 1984, the hospital's Obstetrics/Gynecology Department has been offering to individuals, couples, and families a service that considers both the family and reproductive histories of the women at risk and the social and emotional issues that a diagnosis of cancer raises within the family. The process involves three one-hour visits, after which a comprehensive summary of the risk analysis and the issues discussed is sent both to the individuals involved and to the referring physicians. A number of cancer centers throughout the country are offering risk analysis, following both Kelly's model and other models.

Indeed, the NCI group consider their model as a still-imperfect product of today's limited knowledge. They write, "The projected probabilities [in this study] are intended to provide an aid to decision-making, and despite their considerable uncertainty, may serve as a useful complement to clinical experience and intuition. Major improvements could be made if we better understood the risk factors for breast cancer."[39]

Indeed, if all women understood and acted on what we already know about risk, major improvements could occur both in the quality of lives and the rate of saving lives. Women like Abby would understand that they are not doomed. Women like Jeannette would understand that they have not necessarily been spared. And all women would understand that even if we're not sure we can affect the risk of getting breast cancer, we already know enough to considerably reduce the risk of dying from it. The incidence of several major cancers—most notably cervix and stomach—have dropped off precipitously in the past half century because of human efforts. The Pap smear, which identifies renegade cervical cells before they turn malignant, has saved countless lives. Refrigeration, which keeps food from turning toxic through spoilage and has reduced the need for smoking, pickling, and salting, has probably saved countless more. Twenty-eight years after the first Surgeon General's Report on smoking, American lung cancer rates, which surged in the wake of World War II, the period of heaviest smoking in our history, have also begun to fall. And as public awareness of sunlight's dangers grow, we may see a drop in skin cancers in years to come; deep tans have already lost much of their fashion cachet.

## IN SUMMARY

So what should we conclude from our study of risk? That life is full of danger and breast cancer is, as Abby believes, inevitable? To sum up, we know that:

- Risk is a mathematical relationship, not a prediction.
- Risk statements describe the incidence of a disease in a certain population. They cannot foretell the fate of any individual.
- Factors—in addition to family history of breast cancer—known to increase risk of the disease include menarche before age twelve, menopause after age fifty, childlessness, and a first birth after age thirty.

Certainly, no one can go through life without facing some perils. But these days, given the early detection techniques at our disposal, no one concerned about breast cancer need choose between complacency and despair. Rather, for high-risk women, and for all women, the best choice is vigilance and hope.

# III

❦

# Meeting the Challenge

# 6

❧

# Changing the Odds

THE LAST section explained the nature of the objective
threat that every high-risk woman faces. Now begins the task
of meeting that challenge. A truly effective campaign, we believe, consists of two parts: (1) vigorous early detection practices to safeguard your health, and (2) a set of attitudes and
skills that allow you not only to pursue early detection but to
live with a feeling of hope, optimism, and control in your daily
life.

In this section and the next, we present the elements of
such a program, developed through our research with high-
risk women. Women who follow it, we believe, will not only
assure themselves of high-quality medical surveillance but also
learn to reduce both anxiety and negative thinking about their
high-risk status, achieving a greater sense of positive mastery
over their lives. And these constructive attitudes—in addition
to improving the general quality of daily life—enable women
to pursue their programs of early detection with much less
distress.

But as in every major campaign, success will depend on
careful preparation. You'll need to get all your assets in place
before you undertake your program in earnest. The three chap-

ters in this section will help you accomplish these all-important first steps, showing you how to apply to your own life both personal insights and the scientific knowledge we've gained in the first two sections. First, we'll present the striking evidence that what you do can markedly affect your chances of survival and may even affect your chances of getting breast cancer. Then we'll discuss the considerations involved in choosing the medical adviser you need to carry out your program. And finally, we'll consider an issue that only you can resolve: the impact of high-risk status on your daily life. Once you've accomplished these preliminary tasks, the final section will present a practical, coordinated program for meeting your physical and emotional needs as a high-risk woman.

We begin with an important question.

## WHAT CONSTITUTES SAFETY?

"If I can remove the breast cancer risk," says Helen, thinking of her pioneer forebears, "I feel I can die at eighty like my grandparents."

She proposes to remove what she sees as the one looming threat to her longevity by surgically removing both her healthy breasts. This dramatic step will, she believes, resolve both her risk of breast cancer and her anxiety about it.

"I envy the woman who does that," Abby says. "She's safe. Nothing else will ever make me safe."

But how realistic is the hope of removing the risk? Can any woman, whether at high risk or not, really make herself safe from breast cancer?

The current state of knowledge can't answer either of these questions. But ask a slightly different question—Can you improve your own chances of surviving?—and science answers with an emphatic yes!

No one, in truth, is ever totally safe from the most common of all female malignancies—not even the woman at normal risk; not even the woman who, because of lifestyle choices, is at lower than normal risk; not even, as we shall see, the one who chooses Helen's solution. But every woman, no matter what genetic endowment she carries, now has a better chance than ever of saving her life and, possibly, of cutting her chances of ever getting the disease in the first place. She need only take advantage of today's early detection procedures (which, though regrettably still not perfect, are now the best in history) and of today's most up-to-date advice on lifestyle choices. In this chapter, we'll explain *why* these techniques improve your chances. In Chapter 12, we'll describe in detail *how* you can use them.

## MAKING PROGRESS

No matter what we've said about risk, despite the numbers and studies we've cited, breast cancer still strikes unpredictably. We can't assume, based on what is now known, that any particular person will or won't get it. Statistically, even known risk-group members have a possibility of less than 25 percent. Fully three-fourths of all breast cancers occur in women who lack any known risk factor.

*For all women, therefore, it is very good news that the last two decades have seen major strides in early detection and screening. These advances may be our current best bet for saving more lives.*

This situation represents a big change in both attitudes and technology. More than fifteen years ago, First Lady Betty Ford became a first lady in another sense: the first world figure to go public on the eve of her mastectomy. Shortly afterward, Happy Rockefeller, the vice president's wife, followed suit. That two such famous women revealed that they had a disease that until then was largely kept secret galvanized millions of less prominent women to pay attention to the threat. Overnight, breast cancer became a respectable topic of conversation.

As Mrs. Ford had her surgery, her countrywomen clamored for appointments at the inadequate mammography facilities that then existed. And mammography itself has changed since then from an awkward and fairly inaccurate encounter between relatively few women and some very large X-ray machines, to a refined, accurate, and safe procedure done routinely on millions. Clinical breast exams and self-exams have also gone from taboo to tabloid as celebrity survivors and national magazines proclaim the need for regular breast cancer screening.

That need remains as pressing as it was during the Ford administration. As we mentioned in Chapter 5, *during the last fifty years, the death rate for women at each of the stages of the disease has not changed significantly.*[1] *A woman diagnosed with metastasized breast cancer today is not much better off than she would have been a generation ago. What can save lives now is our increasing ability to find tumors before they have a chance to spread.*

When breast cancer is found before it reaches the lymph nodes, a woman's chances of surviving five years are greater than 90 percent. But her five-year chances fall to 69 percent once malignant cells spread to the lymph nodes, and to 19 percent if they reach more distant organs. Thanks largely to public awareness, however, 60 percent of today's tumors are discovered in the node-negative stage (before the nodes show any involvement)—up from 50 percent a decade ago.[1] That's over 14,000 women a year who have a much better chance of surviving the disease.


## FINDING TUMORS

How to find cancers early enough to make a difference? "The mammogram is one way of seeing the breast tissue,"

Eleanor says, "and the hand is another. That's what my father told me. He's an old-fashioned physician. You need them both, he says, because the one doesn't substitute for the other. Each can see things that the other can't."

Doctors have long suspected that Eleanor's dad was right, and now research clearly backs him up. The best strategy, recent studies show, combines the three "-ams": clinical breast exam, self-exam, and mammogram. The Canadian National Breast Screening Study, conducted in the 1980s, involved 90,000 women aged forty to fifty-nine and found that competent and well-trained nurse and physician examiners can identify breast cancer 80 percent of the time. Modern mammography is accurate 90 percent of the time.[2] A study conducted by the Health Insurance Plan of Greater New York between 1963 and 1986 found that, without mammograms, 30 percent of breast cancers wouldn't have been detected when they were; without clinical exams, 45 percent would have gone undetected. Together, these two methods accounted for 75 percent of detections.[3]

Meanwhile, in the 1985 Swedish Mammography Screening Study, which included 135,000 women aged forty to seventy-five, the survival advantage of regular mammograms was also clear. Over a seven-year follow-up period, women over fifty who had regular mammograms experienced one-third fewer cancer deaths than those who did not.[4] On this side of the ocean, that would add up to tens of thousands of lives saved every year if everyone in this country followed established standards. The Breast Cancer Detection Demonstration Project, conducted from 1973 to 1982 with twenty-nine centers and 285,000 women, showed mammography techniques even better than those in the Health Insurance Plan study. Over the nine years of this study, mammography sensitivity was 71 percent, while clinical breast exam sensitivity was 45 percent. Breast self-exam was most sensitive between the ages of thirty-five and thirty-nine, with a 41 percent tumor discovery rate, and least sensitive in women between sixty and seventy-four, who discovered 21 percent of tumors. Screening with clinical breast exam and mammograms was least sensitive for women between thirty-five and thirty-nine, with a 60 percent tumor detection rate, and most sensitive for those between sixty and seventy-four, with an 81 percent detection rate. Mammography was found to be 91 percent sensitive to breast cancers in women forty to forty-nine years old, and 92 percent for women fifty to fifty-nine.[5]

After years of debate, all the major cancer organizations in this country have agreed on breast screening standards. According to the most recent (June 27, 1989) guidelines supported by eleven major medical groups (including the American Cancer Society, the National Cancer Institute, the American College of Radiology, and the American Academy of Family Physicians), at a minimum:

- All women with any signs or symptoms of breast disease should have mammography as well as clinical breast examinations as often as needed, regardless of age.
- All women should have a baseline mammogram between the ages of thirty-five and forty, whether they have symptoms or not.
- All women between ages forty and fifty should have a physical exam annually and mammography every year, or at most every two years.
- All women over fifty should have both a physical exam and a mammogram every year.[6]

The American Cancer Society also suggests that asymptomatic women from twenty to forty have clinical breast exams every three years.

Keep in mind that these are *minimum* standards for

women with no special symptoms or risk factors. Clearly, if you face a higher risk, you will need more frequent medical attention—twice a year or even more often. A doctor *knowledgeable about breast cancer* is your best guide to what's appropriate for your particular case, as we'll discuss in the next chapter. For further information, you can also call, toll free, the American Cancer Society at 1-800-ACS-2345, or the National Cancer Institute Information Service at 1-800-4-CANCER.

In choosing the facility where you have your mammograms done, the Public Citizen Health Research Group (founded by Ralph Nader) suggests that you ask about the following:

- Is the facility accredited by the American College of Radiology, which evaluates a center's staff, equipment, and procedures?
- Does the facility perform clinical breast exams and does it provide mammography results to patients?
- Is there a radiologist on site to read the mammogram?
- Does the facility have equipment that it uses exclusively for mammography and does it use low-dose radiation?
- How does the facility guarantee quality control?[7]

But medical attention alone won't provide maximum protection. In addition to the two procedures done at the doctor's office or breast center, the American Cancer Society recommends that, beginning at age twenty, every woman examine *herself* every month. This recommendation has a truly lifesaving potential; *90 percent of breast lumps are first found by women themselves.* Even so, only about a third of American women perform this simple survival step each month, according to a national survey, and fewer than that do it correctly.[8] Why should so many of us miss a chance to protect ourselves? The problem isn't knowledge; more than 95 percent of American women know that they should self-examine.

High-risk women do better; between 52 and 64 percent examine themselves. But even among them, compliance could be a lot better. And a proper breast self-exam involves very specific techniques. We'll discuss them in Chapter 12, along with ways of overcoming the barriers to making a monthly habit of what one doctor calls "the single most important thing you can do to save your life."

## PREVENTION

"But mammograms and breast exams only detect cancer," Ruth points out. "They don't prevent it."

Unfortunately, of course, she's right. As we saw in Chapter 4, no one knows for sure what causes cancer. But as we also saw, scientists are pretty well convinced that lifestyle factors help account for our country's high rate of breast cancer. Therefore, in this chapter, to help you consider whether you might want to change any aspects of your lifestyle, we present the evidence. In Chapter 12, as part of the program for healthful living, we will suggest practical ways you can put changes into effect.

### Diet

Anyone who hasn't spent the last five years in a cave or on a desert island has probably heard that a fatty diet promotes cancer. The tie between a high-fat diet and breast tumors is still far from conclusive, and the possible causes are numerous. But whatever the connection turns out to be, scientific leaders such as NCI, ACS, and the National Academy of Sciences already feel confident enough on the basis of epidemiological studies to have weighed in on the side of reducing the fat in the American diet to 30 percent of calories from the present 40 percent—one of the highest proportions in the world. This kind of drop, the experts feel, would also cut our rates of colon and prostate tumors, which also are among the highest in the world.

Evidence of this link has accumulated since the 1940s, when scientists first noticed that mammary tumors shrank in female rats whose diet contained 10 to 20 percent of calories from fat, but not in those who received 40 percent of calories from fat.)[9] Since then, population studies done in the United States, Canada, Italy, France, and Greece have tied lower rates of breast cancer with very low fat intake.[10] The Japanese, who get a mere 10 to 20 percent of their calories from fat, have one-sixth our rate. But when Japanese women move to this country and begin eating the way we do, their rate rises to match our own.[11]

In addition to fat, obesity itself also raises risk, especially after menopause.[12] The level of circulating estrogens, apparently tied to obesity, appears to make the difference. In one study, women with benign breast disease dropped their estrogen levels by reducing their fat intake to 20 percent or less of daily calorie intake.[13] Interestingly, premenopausal obesity doesn't appear to have the same dangerous effect and some consider premenopausal leanness a risk factor.[14] But those who would rationalize their extra pounds with the thought that menopause is some time off should remember that weight loss gets harder, not easier, with the passing years. We don't know the point during the lifespan when diet has its greatest impact on the breasts, but puberty, when breast tissue is rapidly forming, seems a likely bet.

*Many studies suggest that maintaining a normal weight through a diet high in complex carbohydrates and low in animal and vegetable fats might help women and girls of all ages a great deal.* But can a nation of burger, doughnut, and ice cream fans

successfully make the change to low fat? Given a strong
enough incentive, researchers believe—and what could be a
stronger incentive than saving one's life?—Americans can and
will change their eating habits for the better. The Women's
Health Trial Feasibility Study, conducted at the Fred Hutchinson Cancer Research Center during the 1980s by Dr. Maureen
Henderson and colleagues, followed a group of 1,500 women
aged forty-five to sixty-nine who have a cancer risk 1.4 times
normal because of their family and health histories. They successfully cut their fat intake almost in half—from 39 percent to
21 percent—by reducing fats and oils, red meats, whole milk
dairy products, and eggs.[15]

The Women's Health Initiative, an expanded version of
the Women's Health Trial, should go a long way toward clar-
ifying the effects of factors such as diet, exercise, hormones,
smoking, and menopause on such lifestyle illnesses as cancer,
cardiovascular disease, and osteoporosis. The ten-year, half-
billion-dollar project, conducted by various institutes of the
National Institutes of Health, and coordinated by the new
NIH Office of Research on Women's Health, will be the first
long-term study investigating the relationships between lifestyle factors and women's diseases ever conducted in this country.[16]

North of the border, Dr. Norman F. Boyd and colleagues
at the Ludwig Institute for Cancer Research in Toronto have
been working since the mid-1970s with women who have a
breast condition known as mammographic dysplasia. Like
their American counterparts, these women also learned to reduce fat to 15 to 20 percent of caloric intake and to maintain
that level over time.[17] In a 1988 study, women who experience
severe premenstrual breast pain, swelling, and discomfort re-
ported a lessening of these symptoms when they reduced their
fat to 15 percent of calories and increased their complex car-

bohydrates to 65 percent of calories.[18] As 40 percent of premenopausal American women experience these symptoms, 8
percent severely, this type of study obviously merits expansion. And just as obvious is the possibility that reducing dietary fat could be a viable way of reducing cancer risk.

## Exercise

As we've seen in Chapter 5, levels of exercise may be
related to cancer risk. A study of over 5,000 college graduates
by Frisch and colleagues at Harvard University shows that
women who have exercised all their lives experience lower
levels of all reproductive cancers. Specifically, those women
who played on college athletic teams suffer less breast, uterine,
and ovarian cancers than their more sedentary classmates. For
most of us, of course, it's too late to become college athletes
(although it's not too late to encourage our daughters to participate in sports). But it's never too late to become a regular
exerciser. Whether starting exercise later in life has any bearing
on cancer risk is not known.

Still, because it helps reduce anxiety and increase feelings
of mastery and control, it can play an important part in the
coping strategy of high-risk women. Studies conducted with
college students and faculty, for example, found that vigorous
exercise reduces both anxiety and depression and enables individuals to cope better with emotionally taxing situations.[19,20] Studies done with women exclusively also show
that exercise reduced anxiety and depression and increased a
woman's sense of mastery.[21,22] Dr. John Greist and colleagues
at the University of Wisconsin found running as effective as
psychotherapy at alleviating depression. Running, they believe, helps develop a sense of competence and control that
transfers to other areas of life, as runners see their own power

to change their behavior and improve their appearance.[23] Chapter 12 will describe some practical strategies for starting an exercise program.

## Alcohol

"My mother was an alcoholic," Jane recalls. "I always wondered if that had something to do with her cancer."

Research suggests a definite possibility. Like the fat link, though, a tie between alcohol and breast cancer is probable, but not yet clearly established.

Women who take three or more drinks a day raise their risk by 40 percent, according to a 1984 study.[24] Three years later, the Nurses' Health study of 90,000 women aged thirty-four to fifty-nine found that women who drank three times a *week* were 30 to 60 percent more likely to develop breast cancer.[25] By contrast, though, the Framingham Heart Study, a large population project that has run since 1948, found no such connection in women having a drink or more a day.[26] A stronger linkage showed up in the National Health and Nutrition Examination Survey of 7,000 women between twenty-five and seventy-four, especially for the younger, leaner, and premenopausal individuals.[27]

Clearly, more research is needed to clarify the relationship between cancer and alcohol and to find the mechanism that produces the effect. *In the meantime, though, improving your odds probably means limiting the amount you drink, especially if you're at high risk.*

## The Pill

"A doctor wanted me to take birth control pills to regulate my periods," Cindy recalls. "I said, 'With my family history, no way am I doing that!' Can you imagine risking cancer for the sake of something like that?"

Is Cindy right? Would the doctor's suggestion have increased her risk?

This question remains controversial, as it has been for the three decades since the Pill was introduced. Most studies have found that, for most women, oral contraceptives neither increase nor decrease their risk. But for women who take them very early—before age twenty and before a first pregnancy—or very late—after age forty-six—the danger does mount.[28]

Concern centers on early users.[29,30] In 1989, Swedish scientists studied premenopausal breast cancer patients born after 1939—the generation who were young when the Pill first became available. They found that extended use before age twenty-five did correlate with higher risk.[31] Keep in mind, though, that these women took the high-dose pills available in the 1960s. The danger associated with today's low-dose varieties is probably a good deal smaller, experts believe.

In addition to early use, long-term use has been found to increase risk in some studies.[32] The Cancer and Steroid Hormone (CASH) study of the NCI, however, which involved 9,200 women at eight centers across the United States, upon first analysis demonstrated negative results. There was no apparent increase in risk within fifteen years of starting on the Pill. But since these women, on average, began at age twenty-six, the study tells us nothing about the Pill's effects on teenagers.[33] Upon reanalysis, however, increased risk of breast cancer was seen in CASH participants who began menstruating at an early age, never had children, and used oral contraceptives for a long time.[34]

So three important questions remain. Do women who start using these drugs very early increase their risk? Do women who use them for a long time? Do composition and dosage make any difference? To find out, we'd need a very large study of women who both started early and continued for many years.

Until science can provide an answer, then, what's a high-risk woman to do? One thing that we now know for sure is that *not* using the pill will not increase risk.

## Hormones

Does hormone-replacement therapy after menopause increase risk. Here again, the research picture is unclear. In the 1970s, studies showed no relationship between the treatment and breast cancer. But studies done in the 1980s, on larger numbers of women who had used hormones longer, showed some relationships. After fifteen years, American researchers concluded, estrogen replacement may account for a relative risk of 1.5 for women who had natural or surgical menopause. Women who had hysterectomy with removal of ovaries but had used hormone therapy experienced a relative risk of 2.0[35]

In 1989 Swedish scientists found that long-term treatment did increase risk slightly, but only if the woman took progestins. Conjugated estrogens had no such effect.[36] So the type of estrogens used and the presence or absence of other hormones clearly influence breast cancer risk. Obviously, we need more studies of large numbers of women to clarify these relationships.

## The Surgical Option

And what of Helen's solution? Doesn't it seem logical that removing the breast would also remove the risk of breast cancer?

It seems that way, but experience doesn't always bear logic out. As Cindy's sister discovered, and as a study at Memorial Sloan-Kettering Cancer Center shows, breast cancer can develop in remaining tissue even *after* the breasts are removed. Of sixteen women who had subcutaneous prophylactic mastectomies (which left some breast tissue intact), three later developed breast cancer.[37] So even this procedure provides no guarantee that a woman is safe.[38]

Still, for some women who have very high risk and very low tolerance for uncertainty, prophylactic mastectomy may be appropriate. But it remains very controversial among physicians. A prominent doctor once told Abby that "you wouldn't be crazy if you did it, and you wouldn't be crazy if you didn't." He, however, declined to advise her one way or the other, and she let the matter drop.

Because mastectomy is major surgery that may not produce the desired result, anyone considering the procedure should have careful medical and psychological counseling.

## IN SUMMARY

So it turns out that Helen can't guarantee living to be eighty years old. But neither can a person from a family free of any trace of malignancy. But every woman, through the decisions she makes in her daily life, can work to lower her risk. To sum up, she can:

- Practice early detection through breast self-exams, clinical exams, and mammography.
- Eat a diet low in fat and high in complex carbohydrates.
- Limit alcohol intake.

# 7

❦

# *Getting Expert Medical Care*

MANY PEOPLE come away from the research studies, numbers, and data in the last two chapters more confused than ever. They want to know exactly what it means to them. Should a woman get out her calculator and try to do risk computations? Should she arrange to go to a center that does mathematical risk assessment and counseling?

Some people answer both of these questions with an unequivocal yes. Putting an exact number on their degree of risk gives them a greater feeling of control, a sense that they know what they're up against. For others, though, the answer is just as decidedly no. Using a number to define their situation strikes them as cold, abstract, complicated—and numbers are simply approximations anyway. For these women, knowing that they face elevated risk is enough. The exact degree, they feel, doesn't matter.

Both of these are valid responses. Which you favor is a matter of personal choice. If you feel that a full risk assessment would give you the security of knowing where you stand, then you could well benefit from having one done. But if you feel that the added numerical knowledge wouldn't be worth the trouble or expense, you can cope perfectly adequately without it. The essential point that applies to every woman is this: *The exact degree of risk you face is less important than your determination to do what is necessary to protect your health.*

One of the most important steps toward that goal is finding a medical adviser or advisers knowledgeable about breast cancer and sympathetic to your personal needs. Then your advisers can help you make a practical assessment of your personal risk and the steps you should take. Specifically, they will help you develop a prevention program including breast self-exam, clinical breast exams, and mammograms, and advise you regarding the frequency of regular screenings.

You may find the combination of qualities you seek either at a comprehensive breast center based at a hospital, with a physician in private or group practice, or in a clinic setting. You may already have a good relationship with a gynecologist, internist, or general practitioner whom you consult for routine breast screenings, and a radiology center your physician recommends for mammograms. Depending on where you live, you may have access to several good choices or only to one or two (a list of breast centers appears in an appendix). When you find the center or doctor right for you, you will have found your most crucial ally in the campaign to preserve your health, as well as a vital support for your peace of mind.

"Whenever I move to a new town," says Emily, who recently relocated from the West Coast to the East, "one of the first things I do is find out who is considered the top breast cancer specialist in the new place. That's the person I want to see."

Knowing you're at high risk means frequent dealings with health-care professionals. Mammograms, breast exams, even biopsies, are—or should be—routine facts of life. But many women find these medical encounters times of high anxiety, accompanied by unhappy memories and preceded by days of fear. Thus, the high-risk woman's dilemma: The very things you must do to safeguard your life and health are the things that another part of you wants to put off or ignore.

That's why your relationship with your medical advisers, be they staff physicians and nurses at a breast center or HMO, or a private doctor in his or her office, is an important part of any practical coping strategy. But as Emily learned the hard way after her latest move, building that relationship may be trickier than it first appears. Choosing a doctor for technical expertise and a big reputation alone won't necessarily guarantee care that meets all your needs.

"I moved here six months ago," she says. "Right after I arrived, I asked around and, based on what people said, I decided to go to a certain breast center. For a number of years I've had a breast exam every six months. So far I've come to the center twice. But I must say that I'm not completely happy with my experience there. And because of that, I find that I'm really quite upset.

"I've come to realize just how much I rely on knowing that I have someone I trust who knows me and will follow my case. I had established that kind of relationship in Seattle with a doctor I trusted a lot. But so far, I haven't been able to establish anything like that here. Everyone tells me that the people at the breast center are the people to see, that they are the top experts in town. But I have real concerns about my experience with them."

And here she makes her most telling point: "I've learned that my peace of mind depends on having that relationship based on trust."

Our research shows that *many high-risk women consider their relationships with the health professionals who monitor their breast health critical to successful coping and their general well-being. They depend on these advisers for much more than straightforward health screening.* Studies tell us that health practitioners can strongly motivate women to adopt effective preventive health behaviors. This requires a consistent approach toward patients that involves:

- Tailoring health information to the patient's needs.
- Monitoring the patient's progress with the program of screening or treatment they have developed together.
- Examining reasons why the patient might not be following a program of care.
- Involving family members in the patient's care when appropriate.
- Communicating care and concern about the patient's well-being.[1,2]

Abby, for example, knows that her doctor helps her control her anxiety.

"Some years ago, when one of my children was a baby, I found a lump," she recalls. "It turned out to be only a cyst, but it took them four days to get that answer. I nearly went crazy waiting. I went in on Thursday, but it was a holiday weekend and the labs were closed an extra day. There was nothing to be done. The doctor had said when he examined me that he didn't think it was cancerous. But over those four days of waiting, I thought I was very frightened.

"The only thing that really kept me from falling into a deep depression over those days was my doctor's optimism— the fact that he had said he really didn't think it was cancerous. If he had said, 'I don't know,' I think I really might have just ended it all there. To me that means that they think it is cancerous and don't want to tell you. That's what they said to my sister before they told her she had cancer.

"If he had said something like that, I don't know what I would have done."

## THE BEST MEDICINE

So the emotional overtones of a medical visit can affect our sense of vulnerability or control. This happened to Emily in her opening encounter with her new town's "top expert."

"I went for my first visit to these people who had never seen me before," she recalls. "They didn't know anything about me except what they had read in my record. But within a first medical visit, they asked me whether I had considered a prophylactic mastectomy.

"I was really appalled by that. It struck me as very intrusive. I answered that the possibility had been mentioned at least ten years ago, when my sister had breast cancer when she was twenty-eight and I was twenty-five. At that time, she had a prophylactic mastectomy with reconstruction of her unaffected breast. And someone had mentioned to her that her sister—me—might want to consider doing the same thing. But I really didn't want to. It just seemed too drastic, too intrusive. I reacted very negatively to the whole idea.

"But here I was in this new city, with doctors who knew nothing about me or how I coped, and right off they asked me about prophylactic mastectomy! I said, yes, I had heard about it, but no, I wasn't interested. I told them I had had a very bad reaction to the whole idea. But I also said that of course I very much wanted to know their reason for bringing up the subject. Was there some change, some new research, some reason they thought this was especially appropriate to me? I had the feeling that they were sort of advocating it. But they responded that no, there was no particular reason. They were just presenting it as an option that anyone in my situation should know about.

"The whole thing concerned me a great deal. I began to

suspect that they didn't trust their own ability to monitor my case properly. Maybe my situation was more severe, my family history more dramatic, than other people's.

"When my sister had the prophylactic mastectomy, the doctors felt it was appropriate because she really had a hard time handling the uncertainty, the ambiguity. But I can live with the ambiguity. I've lived with it for years. So after I'd been through all that, to have people I barely know suggest the operation without even exploring how I cope with ambiguity disturbed me a great deal."

*The emotional tone of the medical relationship is one factor that can drastically affect a high-risk woman's feelings of satisfaction, control, and competence.* This relationship has been shown to determine the level of patient satisfaction. Health professionals can enhance this satisfaction by demonstrating warmth and friendliness, accounting for the patient's concerns and expectations, and clearly explaining diagnoses and programs of treatment.[3] Because Emily suspected that the breast center staffers lacked confidence in their own abilities, she began to lack confidence in her own future security.

But Ginnie, who has attended the same breast center for several years, put a different, and far more favorable, spin on Emily's experience. "One of the things I really like about this center is that they always lay out all the options for you so you can make your own decisions," she says. "I think they feel it is their responsibility. Perhaps they were just trying to make sure that you knew about all of the options, since they hadn't seen you before. I've never known them to try to force any idea on me. For example, I was the one to raise prophylactic mastectomy with my doctor. He listened to me and then said he would show me a film, give me literature to read, and give me the names of people who had it done so I could speak with them. That made me feel very comfortable."

And Evelyn adds, "After I went through menopause, I had estrogen replacement for a while. But then when I went to the center for my mammogram, they were displeased that I was taking it, given my breasts and my history. I said, 'You're not going to take me off estrogen, are you?' And they said, 'Oh, no, we'll make the decision together.' "

*An effective medical relationship usually involves trust, mutual respect, and joint medical decision-making.* But, according to Harriet, another satisfied client of Emily's breast center, it need not involve the kind of close personal ties with all staff members that Emily was seeking.

"I find that I don't have any emotional connection with the doctors at the center, even though I've been coming for several years. But that doesn't bother me. I have other doctors I feel close to. And I feel that I have much more of an emotional connection with the breast center nurses. Any personal relationship I have is mainly with them."

## STYLE AND SUBSTANCE

The key is to communicate and clarify expectations. What do you *expect* from the doctor who monitors your breast health? Can he or she deliver that?

Based on her experience in Seattle, Emily had come to depend on a certain style of interaction. Because of that expectation, she received a message her new doctor probably did not intend to send—that the breast center lacked confidence in its ability to monitor her properly—and failed to receive the one he apparently intended to send—that she should be aware of all treatment options. *In a medical relationship, style is much more than window dressing.* If, as Marshall McLuhan said, "the medium is the message," then in the medical encounter, style can be treatment.

"Some years ago I had a lump," Eleanor says, "and I

think, if it had been serious, I would probably have saved my own life. First I went to my regular doctor, and he examined me and said he didn't think it was anything. But he also said, 'It might be a good idea to have a mammogram.' But he said it just like that, so casually, that I didn't do anything about it. I thought, 'Well, it's not urgent.' But I still felt uneasy, so I went to another doctor, and he also examined me and also said he didn't think it was anything. And he also said, 'Why don't you think about getting a mammogram.' Again, just like that, so casually.

"Well, I didn't get a mammogram. But I still didn't feel right about the lump, so I went to yet another doctor. He examined me and he said, 'Get a mammogram right away.' So I thought, 'Oh, my goodness,' and I did.

"Of course, getting a mammogram was something I did every year, so there wasn't anything unusual about me getting one. The reason I didn't go immediately was that the first two doctors were so laid back, so casual. It's as if they were so concerned not to alarm anybody. But if the first one had said, 'Go now,' I would have gone. And if anything had been wrong, I would have found it so many months sooner. Doctors are not always trustworthy. The way they express things can make such a difference that it can be a disservice."

Abby, too, learned this the hard way. "I had a sort of funny experience the last time I went to the radiologist," she says. "The year before that, she had read the film and said it looked all right. She said there was no reason to consider a prophylactic mastectomy.

"And the next year I went through the same routine. But this time she called me into her office and said, 'You really should consider a prophylactic mastectomy.' And she told me the names of two surgeons. She said, 'This one's good, but is very busy and you might have to wait several months. So maybe you want to go to this other.'

"Of course, I was horrified. I said, 'Why? What on earth's happened? What's changed?'

"And she said, 'Oh, I don't see any changes. Nothing's changed. There's nothing to be panicky about. But I've seen too many cases of sibling cancer lately.' And that's all it was. It had nothing to do with me, nothing to do with what she saw in my exam. But it disconcerted me."

"Doctors are just people," Chris says. "They are working out of their own experience. Nothing had changed in the literature or research, but your radiologist had just seen a lot of sibling cancer in the past few months. It bothered her. That sort of thing must color a doctor's expertise."

And what colors your doctor's attitude may well color your own.

## GOING THE DISTANCE

So the key is finding a medical situation that makes you feel confident, respected, and secure. Martha, for example, has recently made a change. "I've only been to my current breast center once," she says. "I went to another one previously. But I wasn't satisfied with how they intended to track me, so I moved over here."

"Doctors are like anything else," says Jane. "You have to shop around if you're not getting what you think you need."

*Getting medical care that's right for you may take determination and an entrepreneurial spirit. The first doctor you try may not meet your needs.*

Ask Sheila, who's an expert. In addition to her high risk for breast cancer, she says, "I have lupus and another immune condition. I've had chronic conditions for years. I've trooped into so many doctor's offices in my lifetime. But after many years, I've finally learned that you've got to assert yourself. You've got to say, 'Dammit, you're going to do this and if you don't I'm going to go somewhere else.' You've got to insist. You've got to know yourself, know what's right and wrong with yourself. Plop yourself down in the middle of the office and don't move until they do something. Then they do it, and you're right, and they apologize and you go on."

*Getting medical care that's right for you means knowing your own needs and speaking up about them.*

"You are your own doctor in so many ways," Linda says. "You can feel if something's wrong better than anyone else who's checking you out."

"I think sometimes you have to *not* believe what doctors tell you," Ginnie says. "Whenever I take antibiotics, for example, my nails get all soft and peely. The doctor denied that that was possible. But I knew I was right. When I went off the antibiotics, my nails went back to normal. I think a lot of times doctors preclude things as possible because no one's done the research to prove them."

"And sometimes they just don't know about things," Cindy adds. "I was going to a doctor who wanted me to take birth control pills. I refused. I said, 'Not with my family history.' But he just didn't take my risk seriously. So I changed my doctor.

"Now I have a new gynecologist. The first time I went, I told him my story, and told him that I was there for my six-month breast exam. He gave me a breast exam that was hardly an exam. He barely touched me. But he told me to have my mammogram results sent to him. A couple of days later, he called me all upset. He had gotten the films. He said, 'Do you know about your breasts? Do you know that they're all cystic?'

"I said to him, 'I already told you my history. I told you that was why I came to you. I told you that this was my six-month breast exam.' I told him, 'I came to you for a reason.' He said, 'Yes, yes, I see, I see.' It'll be interesting to see if his exam is any different next time."

"Being assertive isn't as hard as it used to be," says Ruth.

"Women are finally taking charge of themselves, instead of letting doctors take over," Sheila agrees.

*Women who take greater responsibility for their own health care enjoy better emotional and, possibly, physical health. And the women who do best emotionally view their doctors as partners in personal health care—partners selected by the patient and retained as long as the relationship remains mutually satisfactory.*

Abby, for example, makes a special need clear when she makes her appointments. "Whenever I have my mammogram, I always inquire when the radiologist will be in the office and then make my appointment for one of those times. That way there's only a ten-minute wait before the films come up and she reads them. Otherwise there's a two-day turnaround and I really suffer with the anxiety of waiting. They're understanding at the breast center and always cooperate so that I can do that."

By respecting Abby's need for a prompt answer, her breast center shows respect for the emotional side of high-risk status. Emily, on the other hand, in her encounter with the doctor, perceived just the opposite. She interpreted the doctor's question as disinterest in herself as a person and lack of respect for the trials she had faced over the years.

Some physicians, unfortunately, lack insight into the emotional side of patients' situations. Because of their training or temperament, these doctors prefer to deal with objective facts. But health professionals who treat high-risk women routinely face the anger, anxiety, and despair that come from being imperiled by one's genetic legacy.

*Medical advisers who deal positively with these challenging emotions can help women mobilize their own resources for effective coping. This will certainly improve women's emotional state and may well help safeguard their health.*

## NARROWING THE SEARCH

While reading this chapter you have probably been evaluating your own relationship with the physician who does your breast screenings. Many high-risk women use their gynecologists and internists for this type of medical care. A personal physician who provides you with competent professional care will:

- Have the proper training in breast examination techniques to monitor women with a family history of breast cancer.
- Be honest about any limitations of his or her training or skills and recommend other doctors when necessary— for example, surgeons to perform breast biopsy.
- Coordinate care with mammography facilities or comprehensive breast centers for special problems that may arise.
- Understand the emotions that arise for high-risk women in relation to breast screenings, and set aside time to allow for expression of these concerns when necessary.

If you are not already working with a physician, you can get referral names from your state division or county unit of the American Cancer Society. Since the cancer society conducts both professional and public education programs, they will have a list of physicians who specialize in monitoring high-risk women.

You might also consider using a comprehensive breast center for regular breast screenings. A Directory of Breast Cancer Centers appears in this book, following the Afterword. But new centers are being established in many places, so the list may not be complete at the time you read it. You may also want to check with your local chapter of the American Cancer Society and the major hospitals—especially the teaching hospitals—in your area.

*We are convinced that breast centers offer high-risk women valuable pluses.* Most important of these is the integrated approach they take to each individual's situation, offering a wider range of services and a greater depth of expertise than many private practitioners.

As breast health specialists, the staff at breast centers pay full-time attention to developments in detection, research, and treatment. They generally have up-to-date equipment as well as radiologists very experienced at reading mammograms.

But even more important, perhaps, centers usually see themselves as allies with their knowledgeable clients. They stress teaching, particularly of the subtleties of breast self-exam. And they offer the opportunity to form relationships with several sympathetic and informed professionals, a valuable source of emotional support. In addition to physicians, many employ nurse-practitioners highly skilled in clinical breast exam and very adept at instruction.

As gathering places for high-risk women, breast centers also offer possibilities for social support, although few have taken full advantage of them. Many of the women who attended the focus groups that formed the basis for this book found the meetings to be valuable and self-affirming. From these meetings arose networks of friends who share both a common challenge and the ability to help each other meet it. After the professional facilitator stopped conducting the discussions, some group members actively remained in touch. Your own local breast center might be able to provide similar opportunities. Even if it doesn't provide formal, professionally led meetings, it may be possible to arrange less formal gatherings led by high-risk women themselves.

A woman who uses a breast center, however, still needs to

maintain a relationship with another physician or physicians for the rest of her health care needs. This requires that the consumer exercise a greater degree of responsibility for coordination than if she were using a single "one-stop" doctor for everything. We believe, though, that the benefits of expert breast care outweigh the possible minor inconvenience of dealing with more than one doctor.

But not all women in this country have access to comprehensive breast centers. Some, for example, live too far from a center to make regular visits practical. And some women may strongly prefer dealing with a private doctor. They may already have established a relationship that they value. They may feel that a specialized breast center simply adds yet another set of names and faces to an already fragmented system of health care, yet another doctor concerned with a single organ. "I'd like to find a center that screens for all kinds of risks," Roslyn says. "By coming to the breast center, I'm protecting maybe 10 percent of me."

In choosing a doctor, don't forget that you, the consumer, are hiring an expert to fill your needs. You have the right to ask about credentials, experience, and attitudes and to select a physician who helps you feel in control of your health care.

## IN SUMMARY

Competent, caring medical attention can be found in a number of settings. We believe that a comprehensive breast center offers a high-risk woman the best array of resources. But if you do not use a breast center, you can also protect your health by finding a clinic or office that gives you both confidence in its technical competence and a sense of security in its concern for your emotional well-being. It need not be "the top expert in town." It may be the same office that does your regular Pap smear and other routine gynecological care. But your choice should make you feel competent, comfortable, and in control.

Health professionals at such a facility will:

- Take seriously your status and concerns as a member of a risk group.
- Do competent exams.
- Monitor your schedule of routine screening mammograms and clinical breast exams.
- Strongly encourage you to practice other preventive health strategies, including self-examination.
- Show openness to the latest research findings.

Then, in partnership with your chosen medical adviser, you can bring your strengths to bear as you cope with high risk. In the chapters that follow, you will learn how to discover those strengths and how to use them effectively to maximize your chances of good health.

# 8

❦

# *The Role of Risk in Daily Life*

WE'VE COVERED a great deal of emotional and scientific ground since this book began. And now it's time to pull it all together and see how it relates to your own life.

But there's one last step before we get there. You need to understand clearly the role that your own experience, your family's history, and the facts of risk play in your own life. And only you can create that understanding. Only you can accomplish the important task of looking inward at your feelings, actions, and experiences, looking outward at your family and relationships, integrating the facts provided by science, and deciding what it all means to you. In this chapter, once again, we'll hear women speaking about their lives. We hope that they will help you to consider your own life and the role that high-risk status has played, now plays, and will play in it. Starting with the next chapter, we'll outline the specific strategies that can help you to cope with the problems that high-risk status creates and to thrive as a woman in charge of your own life.

We have already explored specific ways that women react to the legacy of breast cancer:

- We've seen how a mother's cancer can change the rest of a preadolescent daughter's life.
- We've seen how a mother's cancer can hone an adult daughter's coping skills and strengthen family ties.
- We've seen how a sister's cancer can raise our sense of vulnerability.
- We've seen how the impact of high-risk status can change over time as we pass important milestones in our personal and family lives.
- We've seen, in short, how high-risk status becomes an issue in our lives.

But how big an issue? An intermittent annoyance that arises occasionally? Or a constant terror that intrudes on day-to-day living? Is it one of a crowd of ordinary concerns or does it tower over most others? Are its effects trivial, or does it influence important decisions?

Abby gives one answer: "Breast cancer affects my life 60 percent of the time. Sixty percent of my inner dialogue is about it. It gets in the way of my everyday functioning."

Anne gives another: "I don't think about it that much. It bothers me mainly when I'm doing my self-exams or coming to the clinic for my checkups or mammograms. It's kind of there, but I don't pay it too much attention."

Martha gives a third: "I feel that if I get breast cancer, I'll deal with it then. For now, I've put it on a shelf. High risk is just a possibility. It's not a guarantee that anything will happen."

And Lillian gives a fourth: "I feel I will be a survivor. My mother got breast cancer at fifty-one. Her mother died three months before that. But it doesn't have me worried. I don't worry about it because I come to the breast center for surveillance."

Recognize yourself in any of these answers? If so, you'll understand a good deal more about your approach to risk before this chapter is over. If not, you can still use these stories to help unravel the meaning of high-risk status in your own life.

Abby, Anne, Martha, and Lilian all face a rather similar statistical risk: each has lost a mother to breast cancer. Two, furthermore, have sisters who have survived the disease. But each of them draws a different lesson from the experience, and risk plays four very different roles in their lives. Have you considered the kind of lesson that you draw from your own circumstances? If not, now would be a good time to consider this important issue and your response to it.

Anne, for example, after years of introspection, has tamed her fear into a manageable annoyance.

Martha, descended from generations of "faith people," sees high-risk status as one of the many crosses to be borne through a life that ultimately rests in God's hands.

Matter-of-fact Lilian, the daughter of "practical Germans," believes that the techniques of surveillance and early detection will protect her.

But Abby finds little comfort, neither in theology nor in technology. She feels ill-at-ease in a world apparently devoid of security. Breast cancer has become a metaphor for her life situation, an emblem of her vulnerability in an indifferent universe. In a strange way, she senses, she even *needs* her risk to focus on.

"On a bad day, it's doom and gloom," she says. "On a good one, things may seem more hopeful. But I always seem to be playing that same game, teetering between those two moods, those two possibilities. The game seems to be pivotal for me. It goes on every day. A good game might last a week or two. But I never miss a day of thinking about it. I can sometimes put the bad things out of my mind for a day or maybe even a week, but then the game always comes back. What triggers it? I don't know. For some reason I'll be in an up mood, and then later on I'll be in a down mood. I don't know why."

Abby's last point raises an important issue. Why do people react to the same threat so very differently? Clearly, neither Abby's anguish nor Martha's serenity nor Lilian's pragmatism nor Anne's acceptance arises from an objective view of future prospects. Abby and Martha face essentially similar statistical odds.

But emotional reactions don't arise from logic. Eve, whose mother died of breast cancer, has tried and failed to harness her reason to control her fear. "My reaction doesn't make a lot of sense," she says. "When I have an exam or a mammogram and they tell me that everything is fine, why aren't I overjoyed? It's as if you're so sure you're going to get it that you almost want to get it over with. You have that hanging thing. Sometimes I lie awake at night thinking about it. I try to fight it logically. I've lived with the scenario that if you get a cancer diagnosis it doesn't necessarily mean you're going to die. I do have a logic track. But then there's this other part of me . . ."

*The importance of breast cancer and high-risk status in a woman's life relates more closely to emotional factors than to objective risk. How frequently a woman thinks about her high-risk status indicates the level of threat and stress that it creates in her life.*

Or as Ruth puts it: "How you react has a lot to do with what you're doing in your life"—with how you feel about yourself and what you think is important.

## HIGH ANXIETY

*How* important breast cancer is varies from woman to woman. *Why* it's important varies, too.

"If I didn't have a child," Harriet says, "I could deal with it. I could deal with being at high risk. But to leave my child the way my mother left me . . . So I find myself thinking about what kind of woman my husband will marry after I'm gone—whether she'll be like me. I think about who I'd want as my kid's stepmother. I wonder if it's the same sort of person that he'd choose."

For Ginnie, the responsibility of parenthood weighs even more heavily. "My mother and sister had breast cancer," she says, "and my husband has already had skin cancer. So he's probably even more susceptible to cancer than I am. Now, *I* realize my risk and try to take good care of myself, but he just refuses to. He takes a really casual attitude toward his health. I just can't get him to pay attention to it. I have to force him to go to the doctor. I had to force him, even when he had the skin cancer, when something was obviously wrong. So I don't think I can count on him to be around to raise our kids if something happens to me. I figure I've *got* to survive."

Eleanor's kids are grown now, but for many years her worries centered on them, and on what she was passing on to them both genetically and psychologically. "I've tried not to let my children see my fear of breast cancer after my mother died of it," she says. "But recently I sent my father some pictures of my daughter. He said, 'She looks just like your mother.' That upset me. I wondered, is it fair to tell that to my daughter? She knows how my mother died. Will she feel the same fear that I do? Does that mean my daughter will also have to be afraid?"

For Harriet and Ginnie and Eleanor, high risk means the fear of not carrying out their responsibilities to children, of dying too early to see them into adulthood, or of crippling their developing psyches. But not for Emily. She sees a different meaning.

"I don't think about death that much in connection with breast cancer," she says. "I think more about disfigurement. I think of the issues as connected with continuing to live with it."

And chief among these is her own future happiness. "I'm in my thirties and single and alone. I wonder about my ability to find a man willing to enter into a relationship with me if this is an issue. It raises issues of sexuality, of what it would mean to my ability to sustain a relationship. It also raises the issue of his willingness to accept the risk of getting involved with someone he can lose."

Charlene, a few years younger than Emily, shivers slightly, her mind leaping past the abstraction of genetic risk to the potential reality of losing a breast. "For a woman to look at herself in the mirror, seeing that part of herself removed, it might take something out of her. It might make her feel less of a woman. It might make her feel less attractive. It might make her feel ashamed that she has to be seen by a male that way.

"I know I would feel ashamed. I wouldn't want any male to see me, unless I knew it was somebody who was really close to me, like my husband. I know if I lost a breast it would really do something to me just to see myself in the mirror, to see that empty place and that scar. I know I would get in a state of depression."

"A friend who had a mastectomy told me, 'It makes me half a woman,' " says Irene, a generation older than Emily and Charlene. "I had to learn to joke with her about it. She said, 'You don't understand.' I said, 'I know I don't understand the way you understand, but I understand that saving your life is the most important thing you can do.' "

But Lauren, in her twenties, shakes her head and says

simply, "I don't think I could cope with it. The idea of taking my clothes off . . . uh-uh."

Irene, a widow who nursed her husband through a final illness that lasted for years, sighs deeply. "We're all afraid of losing that sex appeal that men want. You think about losing that sex play that you enjoy. But I tell this to young people all the time: You never know what's going to happen to you. You have to be ready to adjust when things change. My friend was supposed to have gotten married, but after her operation she backed out. I said to her, 'You're not half a woman. If you'd lost one whole side' "—her left hand sweeps down over her body—" 'well, that would be different. If you don't learn to live with it and learn that you can live with it and be a person, then it's going to be a hard road.'

"Breast cancer could happen to any of us. It has to affect both people in the couple. If he knows you have it, he's concerned about your health. Are you telling me that he'd rather you keep something that could kill you if you could let it go? Come on, ladies! We're talking about reality here. We're talking about where people really are in the heart. If it's all in the bed, then forget it. You don't have anything anyway.

"It could happen to any of us. But I'd hate to think that I'd lose my man because I got sick and couldn't perform. If you do, you've got the wrong man. We're forgetting all the things that go along with this thing—for better or worse."

## AS TIME GOES BY

Evelyn, a decade older than Irene, thoughtfully considers her point. After a moment she says, "Holding a man may not always be an issue, you know," she says. "It isn't for me any more. Your attitude toward your body, and in fact your whole life, changes a great deal over time. At different ages, you feel differently about things.

"At thirty, you want to bear children and be alive to raise them. You want to be attractive. Sex and sexual relationships are very important. You have a greater fear of not living, of not getting what you want to out of your life.

"I'm sixty-one now. I don't mean to say that at this age there's no fear of death, no concern, no desire to continue living. Nearly everyone wants to continue living. But it's different now. You've had your experiences, you've done many things, you've seen what life offers, you have less fear of missing out on what it holds for you. Having small children—or wanting to have them—is a great incentive for staying alive.

"But as you get older, these things change. For one thing, sex decreases in importance. I've been through the menopause, and my interest in sex has rather"—she pauses here, and chuckles—"lessened. For a while, though, I took estrogens for hot flashes and it seemed to revive. At that time, too, I happened to take up with a very nice man. But then I realized the risks of taking hormones in my situation, and went off them. My new interest in sex rather withered. I must say that he was puzzled by the change in me." She laughs.

"A seventy-four-year-old friend of mine recently had breast cancer. The doctors asked her if she wanted reconstruction. She told them no. She said, 'I've had all the lovers I'm going to have.' "

From the perspective of greater experience, Evelyn and Irene make an important point. *The meaning of breast cancer risk changes over a woman's lifetime and means different things at different ages.* As Evelyn accurately observed, the possibility of losing a breast profoundly threatens women in their twenties, thirties, and forties. By the fifties or sixties, the need to keep one's breasts may have become less urgent as, in Evelyn's view, sex diminishes in interest or, as Irene says, more fundamental human values emerge.

## SEASONS OF GRIEF

Not only life, but mourning has its distinct seasons. The risk of cancer can mean different things for people at different stages of accepting a loved one's death.

Linda's mother has been gone just over two years. For the first months, her sorrow was sharp. She had frequent anxiety attacks and felt an intense fear of contracting cancer. Both have now abated somewhat, but her own danger continues to fill her mind. "I think daily about how it would be for my kids not to have a mother," she says. "I think of how painful losing me would be for them, because I know how painful it was for me, and I was an adult. My parents were always—we'll be here, we'll live forever. That was a disservice. You can't live life in a bubble, and I don't. I don't hide my children in a bubble. I let them know that I can die."

Sherri recognizes her own past in Linda's sorrow. "I was cancer-phobic for five years after my mother died," she says. "I was afraid that everything I did or ate or didn't do would give me cancer. After a while it passed, but I later found out that my brother had gone through the same thing. Eventually he told me. But it was a couple of years before we could admit to each other just how frightened of cancer we were."

## TRYING TO COPE

A serious threat demands a serious response, a concerted attempt to cope. At the simplest level, a person at risk may try simply to diffuse the worry; at the most complex, to defuse the danger. Abby tries the first approach, with uncertain results.

"My husband has heart disease all through his family the way there's cancer all through my family," she says. "He's as convinced he's going to die of heart disease as I am I'm going to die of breast cancer. Sometimes, if the breast cancer business gets too much for me, I take a sort of vacation and worry about heart disease for a while. It helps let up the pressure. I guess if you're a worrier, you'll just find something to worry about."

But Eleanor and Helen, not content with surface solutions, have adopted strategies that go to the source of their worry.

"I always thought I needed to prepare my children for the possibility they wouldn't always have a mother," Eleanor says. "I decided to raise them to be as independent as possible. Whenever there was a chance to teach them independence, I took it, even though most people might have considered it odd.

"I always tried to armor them, to make them strong. I felt as if I had this big bottle of love to give to them. I believed that if I gave them enough, if I loved them enough, they would be strong and could face anything. I might not be here. I didn't think my husband would have done a good job raising them on his own. I didn't think I could rely on him. I thought they would have to rely on themselves."

For Helen, occupied with the loss of her "lineblocker," the mother whose health stood between her and the danger, the issue has shifted to assuring her own survival against an inevitability. She has decided to take a difficult step for a woman at high risk of breast cancer: removing both her healthy breasts in a prophylactic mastectomy. This procedure is still relatively uncommon and highly controversial, as we saw in Chapter 6. Some experts doubt that it can totally protect a woman from the possibility of cancer. But Helen has made up her mind. For now, let's put aside the question of whether prophylactic mastectomy represents the soundest medical choice and concentrate on the feelings that Helen and others believe motivate them to make this choice.

"Now, with my mom sick, I'm losing my last female family member to breast cancer," she says. "I hate it. I know

I'm going to do something drastic. I can lose my breasts, but I don't want my kids to lose *me. I* don't want to lose me.

"I don't feel I can control the cancer. Myself is what I feel I can control, even if it's drastic control. My breasts aren't part of my positive identity. And I don't feel myself to be at higher risk than anyone else for any other kind of cancer.

"I want to have this resolved. I want to clear myself of worrying about *me.* I don't want my mom to feel guilty. She didn't choose the genes, I didn't choose the genes. I just want to clear my mind. I'm just scared that I won't do it in time."

Abby sighs as she listens. "I envy the women who've done that. They're safe. Only a mastectomy will ever make me safe. My breasts are full of lumps, they don't make good mammogram images. Nothing can be done short of a double mastectomy, and that's such an enormous step."

Emily says, "My sister had bilateral prophylactic mastectomies with reconstruction. She didn't believe in her ability to cope with the uncertainty. She couldn't deal with the ambiguity. To me, it seemed like taking an easy out."

Sheila disagrees. "It makes a lot of sense to me. My mother had breast cancer sixteen years ago. Then my sister had both breasts removed twelve years ago. She had had cystic breasts for years, and then they found some precancerous cells on one side. They told her it was only a matter of time before it turned cancerous. So she had that one off and a prophylactic mastectomy on the other side, too. She had reconstruction and it looks pretty good.

"I can't see dying to keep your breasts. My grandmother and her sister both had breast cancer, and they knew it. But they never got treatment until the very end. But in those days, you'd rather die than lose your breasts. By the time my grandmother went to the doctor, her whole breast was a tumor. In that generation, it was your breasts and uterus that made you a woman. If you lost them, you were not a woman."

Ruth adds, "After her cancer, my sister also had a prophylactic mastectomy. She had all that tissue emptied out. It
always struck me as a smart idea, a wise idea. Until the operation she went right on making lumps. She was always going
in to have them checked. She's always so anxious, having the
appointments, going in, waiting for the results. Why have all
that stress?"

## OTHER WORRIES

But for some high-risk women, breast cancer does not top
their list of worries and concerns. Even though they recognize
its danger to themselves, they find either that the possibility of
breast cancer does not loom inordinately large in their consciousness or that some other threat looms much larger.

"I don't think in terms of a prophylactic mastectomy,"
Roslyn says wryly, "because I can't take out my colon, my
stomach, my skin . . . What's the use of worrying so much
about one thing when I feel like I'm surrounded by cancer?
There's so much of it all around me. I work at a school, and for
a while last fall, it seemed as though every two weeks someone's parent was dying of cancer. My mother died. Two weeks
before that, my principal's father died. And then two weeks
after that, I heard from my PTA president about one of our
moms, who's in very bad shape with cancer. And it's not all
breast cancer. It scares me that I can't see the moles on my
back well enough to check them every day, that I can't check
my pancreas and my lungs. I feel at high risk for cancer, but
not for breast cancer in particular."

Judy makes the case more graphically. "I don't worry
much about breast cancer. My worry about my body is all
concentrated between my belly button and my crotch. That's
where my angst is. I think all my suffering and pain will be in
there because I have ulcerative colitis and very large fibroids."

And Ruth, in her blunt way, asks: "Why should I be particularly worried about breast cancer? My sister had it, but my mother didn't. She died of pancreatic cancer. Shouldn't I be just as worried about that? Is breast cancer the only thing that we should be worried about as women?"

## COMING TO TERMS WITH RISK

But accepting the risk doesn't mean letting high-risk status rule your life. Sherri has moved from fear to equanimity.

"My mother had no high-risk factors," she said, "but she still died of breast cancer. I, on the other hand, fit into many high-risk categories. Besides having my mother, I had kids late. I'm overweight. And I'm Jewish. We have a higher rate.

"I'm thirty-two and I have a two-year-old son. I've wanted and thought about a second child. But should I have another one? I'm getting closer to the age when my mother died—fifty-two. Then I think, if I wait any longer before I have another child, maybe I'll only know him for ten or eleven years. I'm always thinking, maybe I should have had a child sooner. I think, what a shame I didn't have a kid at twenty-six. But that's ridiculous. You don't run your life that way. You don't have a child because of something like being at high risk. I wasn't ready at twenty-six. I can't make myself crazy in the present because of what might happen ten years from now."

Sheila has a special reason to have come to terms with the risk of illness. "I have lupus as well as being at high risk for breast cancer. I've lived with medical issues for most of my life. And I've learned that you have to arm yourself with all that you can arm yourself with. But you can't let the fear run away with your life. If I did, I'd have nothing left. I'm not afraid of dying. I just live every day. If I get cancer, I'll deal with it when it comes. I incorporate a lot into my daily life, because I have to. The secret is that you just go on."

Chris drew a similar conclusion from her sister's illness. "My sister died of breast cancer, despite doing everything she was supposed to do to fight it. I think the healthiest thing for me is to take precautions, but not let it take over my life."

## IN SUMMARY

So how important is risk in your life? How important *should* it be?

Only you can answer the first question. And the second one has no single answer. But we do know this:

- Different women feel very different levels of concern.
- Levels of concern change with time and changing circumstances.
- The more you think about breast cancer, the more emotional stress you probably feel.
- The level of stress you experience is unrelated to the level of objective risk.

We've also seen how some women attempt to cope with their worry—using techniques that range from the self-defeating—Abby's attempt to worry about something else—to the highly effective—Lilian's and Martha's methods for simply turning their worry off. Perhaps you use some of the same techniques that these women do, or perhaps you have found others that work for you.

But one thing is certain: However she does it, it's vital that a high-risk woman becomes aware of and understands her feelings about breast cancer. Women who feel great distress are less likely to follow effectively the early detection practices that can save their lives. In the section that follows, we'll explore a full range of coping strategies that work for many women. We'll start with cognitive techniques that help you investigate your thoughts, anxiety, and fears. Then we'll go on to specific methods of early detection, diet, and exercise. Using these techniques, we'll help you construct an individual coping program for safeguarding your emotional and physical well-being.

# IV

❦

# *A Program for Successful Living*

# 9

❦

# *Learning to Cope*

BREAST CANCER'S not so much an issue of dying," Emily says, "as an issue of continuing to live."

Or, more exactly, of finding how to live with the ambiguity and anxiety it produces, while carrying out the measures essential to preserving your health. All the women in this book share this challenge. Each has devised a method to meet it.

But, as we've seen, some of the methods work much better than others. Some individuals feel a great deal of distress—anxiety, fear, guilt, depression—about their high-risk status. Some skip the health measures that are their best hope of safeguarding their health.

But others experience much greater hope, confidence, and competence—a general feeling of mastery over the important issues in their lives, including high-risk status. And they combine this upbeat attitude with health practices that take full advantage of today's increasingly powerful technology. Our research clearly shows *women who cope successfully with high-risk status have mastered specific coping skills* that allow them to safeguard their health and also maintain a positive, hopeful, confident attitude toward their health and their lives in general.

The elements of successful coping are not mysterious. In the last couple of decades, psychologists have made important strides in understanding what good coping involves and how individuals can learn to apply these techniques. Now it's time to begin learning these skills.

## THE SCOPE OF COPING

The first step toward effective coping is understanding the nature of the challenge you face. *High-risk women must deal with two distinct but related problem areas: their objective physical risk and the feelings it engenders. More precisely, you must simultaneously cope on two different levels, the medical and the emotional.*

Individual women, as we saw in the last chapter, appraise high-risk status in different ways. Some—particularly those who have both mothers and sisters with the disease—see it as a serious threat that occupies a good deal of their emotional energy. Other women feel anxious only at particular times that bring breast cancer specifically to their attention: when a mammogram or examination is due or when they or someone close to them has a breast problem, like having a tumor that needs a biopsy. Some who cope effectively even see high-risk status as a challenge that they meet through an active program of early detection combined with good diet and exercise habits.

And we must remember that anxiety is not altogether a bad thing. Research has shown that anyone attempting to maintain a health program needs a certain amount to provide motivation. But it must be neither too little nor too much. When people feel either too complacent or too scared, they simply don't follow through. Obviously, then, a woman's attitude toward her legacy of breast cancer to some extent predicts her level of commitment to early detection and prevention. Our own research at Georgetown, as well as that of Drs. Kathryn Kash and Jimmie Holland at Memorial Sloan-Kettering Cancer Center in New York, shows that women who feel moderate anxiety are more likely than those who feel high anxiety to have regular mammograms, clinical breast exams, and breast self-exams.[1,2] Psychological support programs can help high-risk women reduce their distress, encouraging them to increase the regularity of their breast screenings and the likelihood of early detection. Therefore, the social support that breast centers can provide promotes regular screenings because it helps reduce anxiety to manageable levels.

## CHOOSING A STRATEGY

Women who cope well employ—often consciously—specific strategies against specific difficulties. They use *problem-focused coping strategies* to zero in on the demands of their objective situation. And they use *emotion-focused coping strategies* to control their emotional response to that situation. Psychologists Richard Lazarus and Susan Folkman first identified and described these two coping strategies in their cognitive-phenomenological theory of stress and coping.[3,4] Most people combine both strategies in their reaction to any stressful situation, but Folkman and Lazarus found that we tend to emphasize problem-focused techniques in situations we believe we can change and emotion-focused techniques in those we believe we cannot. We're likelier to use problem-focused coping to deal with problems arising at work, for example, than we are in situations like high-risk status, that involve our health.

Because anxiety is so much a part of high-risk status, in fact, good emotion-focused coping that controls distress is a key component of effective prevention. *A complete early detection regimen means confronting the reality of high-risk status. Effective early detection, therefore, also requires controlling and overcoming the distress that may arise from frequent thinking about the possibility of breast cancer.*

To accomplish this control, individuals use a variety of emotional techniques, combining them to match the circumstances. Many, for example, practice what psychologists call positive reappraisal; they strive to find positive meaning from their experience.

"I feel that I'll be a survivor," Jeannette says. "I take very good care of myself."

"Through this I feel a special closeness with my mother, and a sisterhood with all women," Anne says.

Eleanor goes so far as to suggest that "we who've lost our mothers fairly early share something special. It's that good, loving feeling that we have about our mothers. In many of my friends I see that feeling destroyed."

The question of interpreting experience is crucial to successful coping and is far more complicated than it appears at first glance. In chapters 10 and 11 we'll discuss it in detail and learn specific skills that lead to constructive interpretations.

Another important coping approach is seeking social support from friends, family, medical personnel, and others. "Support gives you strength," says Martha, a member of a large, close family. "You need to be able to talk about what's going on with you. I feel great sympathy for those who are alone," she said to Cindy, who had just expressed her fear that she might end up having to face breast cancer on her own, after her husband had left her and her mother and sister were dead. "I feel that if you needed it, I would take you home and take care of you."

Sheila, though, finds friends more comforting than family. "With your friends you can say anything," she says. "But with relatives—well, they tend to get too upset."

The type of support that may be most helpful is a group of women who are in similar situations regarding high-risk status. During the focus group sessions, many participants commented on the excellent and comforting help the discussions provided. These exchanges allowed women to share information and to perceive themselves as members of a larger group, the sisterhood of high risk. As we mentioned in the last chapter, a local breast center may be able to help you find or organize such a group.

Women who cope well also report that they are able to control their anxiety and distress by temporarily detaching themselves from their situation. Only a few women, for example, feel distress about their high-risk status all or even most of the time. For most, the anxiety tends to emerge, predictably enough, when it's time for a mammogram or exam, or when they feel a new lump or a new pain, or when a friend or relative has breast symptoms or a cancer recurrence. Between times, successful copers, though it may seem counterproductive at first glance, may take a vacation from the reality of high risk.

"I don't think about it most of the time," Anne says.

"I put it on a shelf," says Martha.

They concentrate on other, more satisfying aspects of their lives. They keep themselves busy with other interests. They wish their situation were different. Even Abby, who feels a very high level of distress, accomplishes this, as you'll remember, in her own fashion. "When I get tired of worrying about breast cancer," she says, "I spend some time worrying about heart disease." Even this strange and stressful tactic provides her some comfort.

## PROBLEM-FOCUSED COPING

In addition to dealing with emotions, of course, high-risk status also entails a major objective problem, dealing with physical risk of breast cancer. Here, women who cope successfully use the traditional strategy applicable to all successful problem solving: developing a realistic plan of action. The first part of this plan involves defining the problem in a way that enables the woman to personally affect her solution; that is, "I am at high risk for breast cancer," rather than "I will certainly die of cancer." This second statement is not amenable to the same sort of solution.

The next step is gathering information and generating alternative solutions ("I will enroll at a breast center for regular surveillance" or "I'll get exams or mammograms when I think of it"). A successful coper continues to gather information and weighs the solutions according to their costs and benefits ("Regular surveillance is relatively nonintrusive and has been shown to lead to earlier detection and higher survival rates"). Finally, she selects an alternative ("I'll enroll at a breast center"). And she takes action ("I'll read the list in the appendix, select the one nearest me, and call for an appointment today").

The *fact* of high-risk status can't be altered, so effective problem-focused coping involves changing those aspects of the problem that can be altered: improving the quality of early detection and adopting the personal habits associated with lessened incidence.

Implicit in problem solving is the fact that an individual has taken responsibility for finding a solution. That doesn't mean that she has taken *blame* for the problem's existence; no one can possibly be blamed for high-risk status. But she has accepted two propositions: that what she does can make a difference and that she will take active steps, using her own effort and resources, rather than waiting passively for something to happen.

Suzy Szasz, who suffers from the chronic disease systemic lupus erythematosus, draws this distinction beautifully in her book *Living with It: Why You Don't Have to Be Healthy to Be Happy*. To be sure, life with a disease is quite different from life with the threat of one. But if you substitute "high risk" for "chronic illness," and "risk status" for "disease," you end up with a philosophy of life that can serve everyone. Anyone with a chronic illness, she writes, "must recognize that while he is not responsible for his disease, he is responsible for its management. In a sense, this makes living with a chronic illness not very different from living without one: For everyone, healthy or sick, living competently requires assuming maximum responsibility for one's life."[5]

A third approach to coping combines emotion-focused and problem-focused techniques to actively change the situation—like Helen and her proposed prophylactic mastectomy. Although such a strategy often contains elements of risk, it may be very appropriate and reflect good decision making for certain individuals.

By this time, we hope that you've begun thinking of your own most vulnerable times, when your distress about high-risk status is greatest, so that you can begin thinking of ways to prepare for them and protect your peace of mind. Ginnie, for example, invented a special regimen that she follows before each mammography appointment. "First, I imagine the worst—that I will get a bad result, and then I think of what I would do in that situation. Then, just before I go, I listen to a relaxation tape and do relaxation exercises. My husband helps me do them when he can."

So far we've seen lots of examples of productive coping. But there are some strategies that we—and effective copers—would actively avoid. Permanently distancing oneself from a problem and denying its existence may superficially resemble the escape and avoidance techniques that we've just described, but it has a different and very pernicious effect. Good copers may try to escape periodically, but they never detach themselves from the objective problem or minimize its importance. They always "own" the problem in the sense that they accept responsibility for finding ways to cope. They understand that only vigilance will protect their health.

But they refuse to "own" the problem in the sense of accepting any blame for its existence. A genetic fact cannot be anyone's fault or failure. The only failure for which a good coper takes responsibility is the failure to do what can reasonably be done to assure her physical and mental well-being.

# 10

❦

# *A Program of Self-Help*

I BELIEVE I'll get breast cancer," say Abby and Lilian in exactly the same words. "It's only a matter of time."

Then Abby adds: "Nothing can be done to prevent it."

And Lilian adds: "But I come to the clinic on a regular schedule, and I believe they'll catch it early."

Who has the better chance of surviving breast cancer should it come?

You might think that the correct answer is "neither," because ideas probably don't exert very much influence on the genetics of our cancer cells. But the right answer is Lilian. Her ideas may not affect her cells, but they affect her actions. And those certainly affect her health.

Both women, of course, start from a false premise. Breast cancer is not inevitable; the great majority of high-risk women never develop it. But Lilian adds to the equation something that can further improve her odds: She believes she can control her future.

We all know the ordinary definition of control: "the authority to direct or regulate," says Webster's; in practical terms, the ability to regulate outcomes. But Lilian's sense of control is not based on any objective or proven ability, only on her *belief* that she can affect what happens to her. Psychologists recognize that control, to be effective, need not be demonstrated or even real. What empowers an individual is her *perceived* control over negative events.

Psychologist Suzanne Thompson has identified the four factors that empower an individual to control a situation:[1]

1. Ability to use behaviors to take charge of a threatening event (behavioral control).
2. Thinking ability to reappraise the threatening event (cognitive control).
3. Information about the situation or event (information control).
4. Beliefs about the ability to control an event that was not successfully controlled in the past (retrospective control).

We have designed a program of self-help that equips you for success in each of these areas. The chapters of this section will teach you the specific skills you need to achieve the kind of control that will increase your peace of mind and reduce your distress about breast cancer. As you've probably noticed, these skills include both emotion-focused and problem-focused coping methods. Our program consists of four elements:

1. Effective early detection (regular mammograms, clinical breast exams, and breast self-exams), which are explained in detail in Chapter 12. This provides behavioral control.
2. A set of cognitive and relaxation techniques (explained in this chapter and the next) that put you in charge of your thinking, feelings, and reactions concerning your high-risk status. This provides cognitive control.

3. Up-to-date information, provided throughout this book, on current research into ways of reducing your risk, particularly through diet and exercise. This affords information control.

4. Help in understanding your responses to the breast cancers in your family, also provided throughout this book. This affords retrospective control.

Women who follow this program, our research shows, achieve a greater sense of mastery and competence in their lives, which also, as we've seen, permits them to practice effective early detection. (And that, in turn, further increases their confidence.) As you've moved through this book, considering your own experience, feelings, and family history, as well as learning the facts about risk and risk factors, you should already be well along on the third and fourth components of the program.

## THE POWER OF BELIEF

Basic to our program is Lilian's secret weapon: the belief that you can succeed, or what psychologists call a sense of *self-efficacy*. This concept, first defined by psychologist Albert Bandura, concerns people's *judgments* about their abilities to perform a given task. It has little to do with their objective level of skill, but with their *beliefs* about their capacities.[2,3] Do you, for example, *believe* that you could learn to figure skate or play the violin, even if you've never tried? Obviously, you wouldn't get very far toward a figure eight or an arpeggio if you decided that you lack the talent, balance, musical ear, or whatever. And just as obviously, you'd practice hard—and probably make good progress—if you were convinced you could succeed and received encouragement from those around you.

In just the same way, what you believe about your abilities to cope with high-risk status will influence both how you think and how you act. Your beliefs can either encourage or discourage you to persevere with early detection and other health practices; they can increase or decrease the stress, anxiety, and depression you feel during a breast crisis, either your own or a relative's.

*In fact, developing a feeling that your actions can affect your future is probably your most powerful means of coping with the threat of breast cancer. It is basic to both problem-centered and emotion-centered coping.* The threat you face is most decidedly not just in your mind. But that's where you may find your most powerful defense.

Your beliefs about your abilities influence each stage of developing and carrying out your personal program of self-help, which should include regular mammograms, clinical exams, and self-exams; modifications in diet and exercise habits; and a number of techniques explained in this chapter and the next that can help control anxiety and depression. If, for example, you believed "It wouldn't do any good" or "It's all too complicated" or "I'll never be able to stick with it," you wouldn't even consider adopting either a sound screening program or changes in your diet and exercise habits. But once you're under way, once you've seen yourself start and stay with a program, the experience of success will convince you of your personal effectiveness. It will increase your willingness to continue and lessen your anxiety and fear. This simple fact, that success produces confidence and confidence reduces distress, is the basis of the program developed at the Georgetown University Comprehensive Breast Center and of the program we are recommending to you.

Some features of the program may have visible results. Reducing dietary fat and exercising regularly, for example, could lead to a slimmer figure. The cognitive and relaxation techniques to control anxiety could lead to a more relaxed outlook in other areas of a woman's life. But the early detection portion has a problematic feature: *Putting it into practice requires a lifelong commitment to preventive procedures—mammograms and breast self-exams—that you may not want to do. And if successfully done, these practices produce no obvious results.*

It's just the opposite of the way incentives usually work. Ordinarily, when we do a good job, we see positive results, we get compliments, we reach desired goals. But your campaign against breast cancer won't offer many clear-cut rewards. It's rather like buckling up your seatbelt every time you get in the car to protect yourself against the accident you hope will never happen. When you put the early detection program into effect, here's what will happen to signal success: absolutely nothing. Under the best-case scenario, month after month, year after year, not a single errant cell will turn up on the X-ray plate or under your own or your physician's hand. Decade after decade, you will not develop cancer, and you'll never be sure that your prevention efforts had a real effect. Or, in the second-best case, a small growth in early stage I will reveal itself in a mammogram or breast exam. Prompt treatment will remove it and there will be no spread.

And so we can see clearly why Lilian copes better with high-risk status than Abby: Lilian *believes* that her efforts give her some control over her future and therefore she will probably *persevere* in those efforts longer and more faithfully than someone who does not. Regardless of whether her belief is scientifically accurate, it encourages her to keep up her regimen. It also helps her live to the fullest while doing so.


## REAL EFFECTS

Researchers have seen the results of such positive beliefs in many kinds of health practices. They've concluded that people who feel they can succeed do better than those who harbor doubts when it comes to quitting smoking, maintaining an exercise plan, controlling drinking, and consistently using birth control.[4,5,6,7] The same goes for weight loss.[8] People with high self-efficacy—those who strongly believe in their ability to persevere and resist returning to their old ways—fare better than those with less faith in their own powers. Self-efficacy is one of the best predictors of a person's ability to change her health practices and maintain this change.[9] Success requires that an individual has made a voluntary decision to change her behavior. In the case of high-risk women, this means deciding to learn about, adopt, and maintain regular breast self-exams, clinical breast exams, and mammograms.

The meaning for high-risk women is clear. Anyone with a chronic health issue that requires continued commitment to health practices needs to believe that she can make a difference. A diabetic who know that regulating diet and taking insulin will prevent comas, an epileptic who knows that taking medication will forestall seizures, a heart patient who believes that low cholesterol will lessen the risk of another attack, someone with high blood pressure who knows that daily medicine can prevent a stroke, a sufferer from gum disease who knows that careful flossing and brushing can help her keep her teeth—all these people know what they need to do and will continue, year after year, to do it.

And there's another, equally important, benefit. In prevention, says Linda, who has rigorously followed a low-fat vegetarian diet for almost a decade, "the issue is control—even if we don't know what is actually preventive." And that's especially true with a problem like high-risk status, which is both amorphous and permanent. Linda, for example, has read enough to know that lowering fat may lower cancer risk. Maintaining a low-fat, vegetarian diet makes her feel that she is effectively controlling at least one aspect of her problem. And her success at taking control in one area of life gives her the confidence to consider taking charge of other parts as well. As was shown in a study of women who successfully follow an exercise program,[10] *people who have a high degree of self-efficacy concerning a health problem feel greater mastery, both over the problem itself and over their lives in general.*

## LEARNING SELF-EFFICACY

Sounds good, doesn't it? And it is. A feeling of mastery can get you into what scientists call a positive feedback loop. You believe you can do something effective about a problem. And every time you successfully do that thing, the good feeling you get strengthens your confidence in your abilities. And that, of course, encourages you to do it again.

But how do you start? Because a key to self-efficacy is the experience of success, we're going to help you to write a *personal behavioral contract* that will allow you to define success and then to measure it and reward yourself. As we've already mentioned, there's no good way to measure success at early detection. But you can measure your success at *following the terms of your contract.*

Setting up a plan that allows you to do this involves four steps. First, you'll clarify and define your expectations. Second, you'll specify particular goals. Next, you'll select ways of rewarding yourself for following through, and finally, in three months, you'll take stock of your progress and make any changes that will help you do even better.

All this may seem obvious, but there's great value in going through the process step by step. We recommend that you actually write down your agreement with yourself. You can do that by filling in the form on pages 160–161. (We recommend that you first make photocopies and fill them in rather than writing in the book; you'll want to keep the original clean so

## BREAST HEALTH CONTRACT

I, _____, agree to begin or
    (your name)

maintain my commitment to:

_____breast self-exams      _____clinical breast exams

_____mammograms      _____low-fat diet

_____exercise program      _____relaxation training

under the following circumstances: _____
(where, when, how often, for what time period)

_____

I will begin on _____ and plan to reach the following
       (date)

goals (stated so that they can be measured; e.g., to exercise
three times a week for twenty-five minutes each time, to practice a relaxation technique for ten minutes each day)

_____

_____ by this date _____

*To help me do this, I am going to:*

1. Make the following changes in my physical and social environment (e.g., place reminder notices for breast self-exam
   in bedroom and bathroom, stock pantry and refrigerator
   with low-fat foods):

_____

_____

2. Control my internal environment (thoughts, emotions, images) by:

_____

_____

3. Use the following methods to chart my progress toward reaching my goal (e.g., food diaries, graphs, charts):

_____

_____

*Reinforcements (supports):*

Reinforcements provided by me (when I keep contract):

_____

How often (weekly, monthly, etc.): _____
Reinforcements provided by others (when I keep contract):

_____

How often (weekly, monthly, etc.): _____
Support person with whom I will discuss how this program is going: _____

*Additional pertinent information:*

1. Baseline information (e.g., how often I currently practice breast self-exam, have clinical breast exams and mammograms; my typical diet for three days; my weekly exercise program; my weekly relaxation training program):

_____

2. Attach charts, graphs, diaries to this contract.

3. Evaluation method (How will I judge my success? Summarize my experience until now and the changes I will make in continuing my program)

that you can use it to make changes in your contract later on.) As you see, in the contract you agree to follow certain health behaviors and then to give yourself specified rewards when you succeed.

Your expectations will play a key role in your success, and only you can determine what they are. To help in clarification, we suggest that you answer this series of questions:

QUESTION 1. *What health behaviors do I want to change and why are these important to me?* A possible answer might be: "I want to practice effective early detection to protect myself from breast cancer" or "I want to do mammograms, clinical breast exams and self-exams more regularly so that I can feel less anxious about being at high risk."

QUESTION 2. *What short-term and long-term benefits do I anticipate as a result of this change?* Possible answers might be: "I expect it will give me a much greater feeling of control every day" and "I expect it will increase my chances of long-term survival."

QUESTION 3. *What needs are being met by my present behavior?* This question requires looking deeply and honestly into your feelings. Some women might say, for example, "Failing to do adequate early detection keeps me from having to confront the reality of high risk." Others might add, "Feeling myself a victim of circumstances relieves me from having to take responsibility for my health."

QUESTION 4. *What needs will be met by changing?* A possible answer is: "I will be better able to deal with my anxiety" or "I will get a feeling of control in my life."

QUESTION 5. *What are the physical, social, and internal barriers to making this change?* Physical barriers might include such things as distance from a clinic. Social barriers might include the inconvenience of going to appointments or the expense of care. But internal barriers are likely to be both the strongest and the most diffuse: anxiety, fear, procrastination.

QUESTION 6. *What physical, social, and internal supports do I have for making this change?* Possible answers: "I can easily drive or take a bus to the clinic." "I have insurance that will cover this care." And especially important social supports may become apparent. "My family members want me to take care of myself" or "My husband will encourage me" or "My friends will be willing to listen to my anxieties before I go for my mammogram" or "My doctor or the people at the breast center will be very supportive." And internal supports emerge as well: "I have the strength to take charge of my life" or "I am very determined when I make up my mind to do something" or "I am an intelligent, informed person determined to safeguard my health."

QUESTION 7. *What skills and competencies will I need in order to change?* Possible answers range from "I need to know how to do an effective breast self-exam" to "I need to know how to control my anxiety." One person might answer, "I expect my professional adviser to provide significant emotional support at the traumatic times of my examinations." A second might say, "I expect technically competent medical care." A third might add, "I expect my doctors and nurses to take my own specific needs into account."

It's important to your success that your expectations be as realistic as possible. Your doctor, for example, may not be willing or able to provide the emotional support you seek. You don't want your disappointment at an expectation that doesn't work out to undermine your confidence in your abilities.

It's just as important to be clear about your feelings on undertaking this program. Are you hopeful? Worried? Scared? Intimidated? Determined? Confident? Does taking definite steps to get control of your high-risk situation make you tense (because now you'll have to think about it more) or enthusiastic (because you're finally *doing* something about it)? These are only a few of the possible emotional reactions women might have. But knowing which one you feel will help you understand and deal with any feelings that may stand in the way of success (more about this in the next chapter).

Now it's time to define specific goals. Here are the ones we recommend:

"I agree to perform breast self-exams regularly and have mammograms and clinical exams regularly as well under the following circumstances: I will do my BSE each month on the tenth day after my period begins or on the tenth day (or any other specific day) of each month if I no longer have my periods. I will have my mammograms as often as my doctor or the breast center advises."

Next, consider your own personal barriers and supports, and plan how you can help yourself comply with the contract. For example, "I will arrange my physical and social environment by telling my best friend about my problem doing BSE so that she will congratulate me each time after I do it" or "doing my BSE early in the morning, before my husband has gone to work, so that he will be with me in case I find anything scary" or "finding a mammography center that is easier to get to than the one I've been using."

You'll probably want to fill in the part about internal environment after you've learned the cognitive and relaxation skills in Chapter 11.

Next, think of some ways to reward yourself for maintaining your program, some that you would give yourself, some that other people might give to you. We suggest that you choose rewards you really enjoy. Every month, after you check off your breast self-exam, for example, you might treat yourself to a special hairdo or a new mystery novel or one beautiful piece of fruit or something just as delicious that doesn't cost a cent: an hour listening to your favorite music, watching a favorite TV show, or walking instead of doing chores. A special dinner or a new scarf, for example, might reward each visit for mammogram and clinical exam. Reinforcements from others might involve their congratulations, or their company on your walk or for dinner. Now write your chosen reward on the contract form.

You'll need a way of tracking your accomplishments: a calendar, chart, or diary where you record each time you do a BSE or have a mammogram or clinical exam. Each time you fulfill one of the terms of the contract—each month you do your self-exam or each day you exercise—you should fill in the appropriate box.

And then, at the end of three months, you will have a real measure of your progress. You will see by the filled-in blanks how well you followed your contract. And your experience will tell how well the contract suits you. You may wish, when evaluation time rolls around, to modify the terms a bit, to change the rewards, for example, or to alter the diet or exercise plan you've established.

So now, we hope, you're well on your way to planning your personal program. And even if you're skeptical, we hope you'll give it a try. And if your own prospects of success don't convince you at first, consider some of the women we've met in this book. A number of them serve as examples to us that ordinary women, women much like yourself, can and do achieve sound emotional adjustments and stick to regimens of good health.

Specific training in techniques will also help lead to success. You'll find it useful to ask your doctor or a staffer at your breast center to clarify any details of your breast health regimen that seem unclear.

And finally, a factor that can greatly affect your belief in your abilities is your own state of mind. Anxiety and depression can falsely convince you that you're likely to fail. The next chapter will tell you how to work with negative emotions when they occur. You'll also see how you can develop the self-support and positive beliefs needed to maintain your program.

## FINDING SUCCESS

As you undertake your program, though, it's important to understand what we mean by success. In dealing with high-risk status, succeeding means taking the best care of yourself that you reasonably can. It doesn't mean falling into the emotional trap that Helen did.

"We gave early detection a try," she says. "It didn't work. My mother did everything she was supposed to, and was still diagnosed with cancer. My faith in vigilance was destroyed. I've completely lost faith in that." And, of course, she's also lost all motivation to persevere over the long haul in her own breast health practices. Doesn't Helen imply that people like Linda are deluding themselves, that the control they feel is nothing more than a comforting illusion, a kind of denial of the unpleasant truth?

Not if you understand it correctly. Control isn't unitary and it's rarely total. Psychologists recognize a distinction that's relevant here, between *absolute control* and *probabilistic control*. This second kind does not guarantee that something won't happen, but it does make that thing less probable. It doesn't control the outcome, but it alters the odds.

As we've seen, regular mammography alone can reduce mortality by 30 percent. Add that to the rest of our detection and lifestyle strategies, and the odds ought to improve even more. Following the program that we've suggested is the way you can improve your odds. You'll know that you've done all that is humanly possible to influence your health. So when

Helen says that "vigilance failed," she means that it failed to do what everyone knows it can't do: it failed to provide a 100 percent guarantee.

Jane takes an attitude that will prove more resilient in the long run. "My sister died despite doing everything she was supposed to," she says. "The healthiest thing for us is to take precautions but not let it take over our lives."

Failure in the context of high risk is not failing to prevent cancer (which is impossible) but failing to do what we can to protect ourselves. And then, as Jane says, going on about our lives. A constructive attitude toward health practices is a balance between controlling what you can and accepting that you can't control everything, between the determination to do all that you can to protect yourself and the refusal to blame yourself for the outcome, which is beyond your absolute control.

Evelyn remembers an incident on a transatlantic airplane flight. "I suddenly became aware that something was wrong," she says. "They didn't announce anything, but I realized that they were dumping fuel. I didn't know that that was normal procedure for lightening the plane. I thought that they were expecting a crash imminently.

"Now, there I was sitting on that plane. I was totally helpless. But even so, I was totally serene. There was nothing for me to do. I didn't pray and I didn't scream. In a situation like that, you give up. What will be will be. Faith is putting things in the hands of God. That's what I did. I put things in the hands of God and I waited."

## IN SUMMARY

In the final analysis, any high-risk woman's ultimate fate is partly in the hands of destiny or genetics or whatever she wishes to call the factors still beyond human control—and partly in her own. She cannot change her genetic endowment or some of the other factors that determine her mathematical risk: when she had her children, whether she was exposed to carcinogens, all other events that occurred in the past. But she can control her future. She can control what she eats and whether she exercises and how often she examines herself, goes for clinical breast exams, and has mammograms. She cannot guarantee her outcome, but she *can* guarantee that she gives herself the best possible chance.

Martha says she comes from a family of "faith people," who trust in God. But she is also a woman of high self-efficacy who knows that, as the old saying goes, "heaven helps those who help themselves." She has aggressively sought out the best care for herself, changing from one breast center to another when she became dissatisfied with the care she received. "There's always something you can do," she says. "I always perceive that there is something you can do."

Once again, she's right. In the next chapter, we begin to specify what those things are.

# 11

❦

# *Cognitive Skills*

Now, with the main elements of your program in place, it's time to learn the particular skills that lead to success. In this chapter we're going to show you how to deal with the negative thoughts and feelings that undermine confidence and self-efficacy. Specifically, we're going to teach the techniques that people who cope well use to reduce distress and gain control over their lives.

That's right: *learn the techniques*. These women may not know it, may not think of themselves as doing anything special, may not consider they're doing anything more than getting by. But in fact, our research has shown that well-adjusted, high-risk women share certain habits and attitudes that help them cope effectively. And it further shows that these habits and attitudes can be learned, and, indeed, *must* be learned by every high-risk woman who wants to maximize her chances of staying healthy.

## LEARNING TO LISTEN

Throughout this book, we've heard women talk about their mothers, their sisters, and themselves; about diagnoses, treatments, and operations; about suffering or triumph. And also about loving support; about resignation, anger, disillusionment, and disappointment; or about generosity, tenderness, serenity, and courage. We've heard about mothers who gave up and mothers who fought valiantly, about sisters who put their faith in God and sisters who lost their faith in everything.

Although we haven't said it in so many words, chapter after chapter we've been listening to women answer these four questions:

- What do you believe causes breast cancer?
- How did your mother or sister respond to the disease?
- What strategies did you use to cope with your mother's or sister's illness?
- What do you feel, believe, and do about your own elevated risk?

These questions don't represent random curiosity, but rather were developed through a large body of research on health issues. We designed them to investigate the beliefs that help or hinder a woman in achieving a positive emotional adjustment to her high-risk status. Each of the women we've heard has revealed:

- Her belief in her ability to affect her health and lessen her danger from breast cancer.
- Her belief in her ability to affect the course of her life.
- Her belief in her ability to cope with breast cancer should it come.

Now it is time for *you* to undertake a difficult but liberating task. It is time for *you* to uncover your own beliefs, to identify the thoughts from the past you may have forgotten.

We will present several questions. We hope that you will take the time to answer them as truthfully and thoughtfully as possible. Think carefully and honestly about your own beliefs. Write them down. When you read them back, you'll begin to see how you've been talking to yourself about breast cancer.

As many of the women in this book have found, *coming to terms with your own relative's breast cancer can help you feel less vulnerable and better able to cope with your risk.* It is, in fact, a major and necessary step toward the positive adjustment that can both enrich your days and help save your life.

Now please answer the following questions:

- What do I *believe* caused my mother's, sister's, or other relative's breast cancer?
- How did I *feel* during her illness?
- What did I *think* as I went through the disease process with her?
- What did I *do* to cope with breast cancer? What did *she* do?

Women who cope successfully with their high-risk status, our research shows, are aware of and understand the feelings, thoughts, and actions that surround their situation. They understand them on two levels: both as historical facts and as emotional reactions. They know that things happened in a certain way. And, even more importantly for their future adjustment, *they understand that they perceived them in a certain way. And that perception has helped determine their present ability to cope.* It is only by exploring your own memories and feelings that you too can identify actual events and personal feelings in response to them.

Nothing can change the fact of your mother's or sister's illness. But if you have destructive perceptions of it, you *can* change those perceptions. You can search for the positive in your family's history, not by ignoring your pain, but by paying new attention to your relative's dignity and strength in the face of adversity, and to your own ability to persevere in the face of the adversity that faces you. And by doing that, you can strengthen your own power to live the life you want to live.

## CHANGING SELF-TALK

At this point, many people might be thinking, "This is simply a pitch for positive thinking." But it is much more than that. It is a method derived from a large body of sound and highly respected psychological research.

In 1955, Dr. Albert Ellis, a psychologist looking into the origins of depression, devised a system he calls rational-emotive therapy.[1] *Events in themselves do not cause the distress in our lives, Ellis said. Rather, our beliefs or "self-talk" about those events contribute to our depression and distress.* For Ellis, it was a process as simple as ABC—letters that he used to stand for important elements in our mental processes.

For every A, or activating event, there exist many possible Bs, or beliefs, thoughts, cognitions, and ideas that interpret that event and put it in context. Those defining Bs, in turn, strongly influence the Cs, or consequences of the event, whether they take the form of feelings, ideas, or actions.

It's easy if you think of it this way:

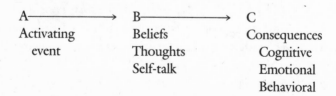

| A $\longrightarrow$ | B $\longrightarrow$ | C |
|---|---|---|
| Activating | Beliefs | Consequences |
| event | Thoughts | Cognitive |
| | Self-talk | Emotional |
| | | Behavioral |

Eleanor's experience with her daughter's portrait provides a perfect case in point. As you may remember, Eleanor sent her father a copy of the photo, and he told how happy he was to receive it because twenty-year-old Holly "looks just like" his late wife, Eleanor's mother.

But this affectionate and well-intentioned comment upset Eleanor greatly. "It frightens me that my daughter looks just like my mother, who died of breast cancer," she says. "Does the physical similarity mean that she also will die of breast cancer? If I tell Holly what my father said, will it frighten her? Will she also worry about getting it?"

The A or activating event was Eleanor's father's comment. The B or belief was Eleanor's assumption that this implied Holly might get breast cancer. The C or consequence was Eleanor's feeling of distress.

Eleanor's response was immediate, spontaneous, and natural. It expressed the emotional reality that defines the situation for her.

But it's easy to think of other ways to interpret her father's remark. Looking back over the incident, Eleanor herself immediately sees one: "I could have thought, 'How nice that Dad thinks Holly looks just like Mom, whom I loved and admired. I hope she'll also grow into just as fine a person.'"

And Ruth offered another possibility: "Your daughter never knew your mother, so she won't think of how she died. To her, her grandmother is a lovely lady of mystery."

Thinking over these alternatives, Eleanor now realizes something more crucial still. *Her first statement caused her distress. The other two do not.* In fact, the other two provide comfort and encouragement.

Thus, for example, for Eleanor's A, her father's comment about Holly's resemblance to her grandmother, there are at least these three possible Bs: Eleanor could surmise that the resemblance implies breast cancer and a life of worry for Holly too. Or Eleanor could feel pride that Holly resembles so admirable a person as her grandmother. Or Eleanor could realize that Holly did not know her grandmother and therefore has no unpleasant associations with her memory. Probably you can think of other possible beliefs as well.

Each of these Bs obviously leads to a quite different C. The first, as we've seen, directly evokes anxiety, worry, and feelings of helplessness in the face of an implacable threat. The second two evoke pleasant feelings of pride and fondness and, possibly, nostalgic and affectionate reminiscences of a deeply loved relative. Thus, *Eleanor's perceptions and feelings about this incident are largely determined by the "self-talk," or active thinking she does about her situation.*

But positive self-talk can do more than turn off distress. It can help change difficult, unsatisfactory situations. Let's consider Laura, who, you'll remember, brought her mother, Mary, home from the hospital and cared for her until she died. If we examine the structure of that decision, we see that it was Laura's positive self-talk that permitted her family to fashion a loving solution to a difficult problem.

Let's go back to the moment of decision, to Laura and her parents in her mother's hospital room. We start our analysis at the moment of the emotionally charged activating event (A): The doctor tells the three family members that he will shortly discharge Mary and that she must go to a nursing home because "she can't be cared for at home." Paul, Laura's father, is the first to express his belief (B); he accepts the doctor's assessment that Mary must enter an institution. Mary even unwillingly accepts that belief, so that she won't "cause trouble" for the family. But she hates the consequence (C) that logically follows, and begins to weep.

Laura now boldly recasts the situation and asserts a different belief: "We can find a way to take care of Mother ourselves." And she moves directly to a quite different and more satisfying consequence: "We're not sending her to any nursing home. We're taking her home."

Next, Laura set out to test her belief—and at that point, it was not more than a belief. She did not actually know whether it was accurate. As the hospital prepared to release Mary, Laura set to work investigating the resources in their community that would let her fulfill Mary's wish. And in the end, Laura's belief proved sound. With the help of a home-hospice agency, with the cooperation of her employer, with the collaboration of her father and family, she assembled the care that Mary needed to spend her last days as she wished, among those she loved in her own home. And Laura and her family avoided the distress and guilt that they would have experienced seeing their mother unwillingly confined to a nursing home.

As you'll remember, Mary spent much of her remaining time composing letters to her friends thanking them for what they had meant in her life. For Mary, even the end of life could have a positive meaning: It provided the opportunity to express love and gratitude. Once again we see the power of self-talk in decision making and determining outcomes.

## THINKING ON THE BRIGHT SIDE

Negative self-talk fosters the fear, anxiety, and depression that trouble many high-risk women. But it's possible to make a more productive adjustment to a difficult situation. Women who accomplish this do not allow negative self-talk to interfere unduly with their lives or distort their moods. They have learned to limit their fear and anxiety in certain situations and at a level that they can tolerate.

Being able to do this means resisting the three major temptations that Ellis believes lead to negative thinking. The first is a tendency to "awfulize" one's situation—to make it worse than it actually is. "There's nothing that can be done," Abby says, for example. "I know I'm going to get breast cancer. It's only a matter of time." She sees no way of getting free of this problem, no matter what she does.

But high-risk status becomes less awful if we see it not as a unique curse but as a normal part of living. "Is breast cancer the only thing we should be worried about as women?" Ruth asks. "My mother died of *pancreatic* cancer."

"It's just another thing that's sent to us," Teresa says.

"We're all at risk for *something*," Jeannette adds. "All of our parents died of something."

High-risk status becomes less awful when we realize that most people would be at risk for some disease if the origin of all diseases were known. It just so happens that breast cancer's family patterns have been intensively studied. As Abby admits, "Heart disease is all through my husband's family the way breast cancer is through mine." The genetic component of heart disease is also well known, as is true of diabetes and many other types of cancer, and the lupus that Sheila shares with her sister. Some researchers also look for genetic bases for Alzheimer's and schizophrenia. Looked at this way, high risk for breast cancer becomes just one of many threats that face individuals, not an extraordinary doom but an ordinary expression of the human condition. Living at high risk becomes normal living.

The second trap, what Ellis calls "I-can't-stand-it-itis," is particularly pernicious for a high-risk woman. Here, the threat dominates her daily existence, reducing the enjoyment her life has to offer. She doubts her own ability to cope with its demands or to tolerate the stress it creates. "I think about it every day," Abby says. "Sixty percent of my interior dialogue involves breast cancer."

A way out of trap number two is what Ellis calls "tolerance." A woman who can tolerate her situation acknowledges that she is vulnerable to breast cancer. She knows that fretting and emotion won't prevent it. But she takes a pragmatic approach, considering what the reality of cancer would be in her life and what resources she would muster against it. She remains mindful both of its dangers and of the strengths that she could call upon to cope with the crisis. Eleanor, you'll remember, worked at teaching her children independence so that they could survive without a mother if need be.

"I'd probably be angry at man and God," Martha says, "but I'd fight."

"I think I'd be a survivor," Lilian asserts.

By considering this terrible possibility concretely, these women make it an integral—but far from dominant—part of their lives. Then they alter their lifestyles as much as they reasonably can to minimize their risk. And, having done all they can, they actively pursue their lives and goals despite a status that cannot be altered.

"I think I'm going to get breast cancer," Sherri says. "In fact, I think I'll probably die of it. But I'm not going to make myself crazy in the present over something that might or might not happen ten years from now."

The third trap is what Ellis calls "damnation," a sense of inescapable doom. Helen, for example, thinks that the only way she can protect herself from breast cancer is with a prophylactic mastectomy. "I really envy a woman who does that," Abby says. "Nothing else will ever make me safe."

Many women who accept the fact of high-risk status as a reality beyond their control feel neither blame for the outcome nor a need to "guarantee" their survival. They recognize that no one can ever be completely safe. This doesn't imply passive resignation, though. Rather, they take control of those aspects of life and health that they can affect—but without the need to be perfect. For some women this may involve prophylactic mastectomy. Their efforts represent a sincere effort to do what is humanly possible—but nothing more—about their situation.

Linda, for example, believes in a strong link between diet and health. For almost a decade, she has maintained a vegetarian household for her husband and three sons. Since her mother's breast cancer two years ago, she has put special emphasis on low-fat foods. "We try to limit desserts," she says, "because they tend to be high in fats. But even so, a couple of times a week we'll have a dessert. People like dessert. There's such a thing as being rigorous, and then there's such a thing as being so rigid you can't enjoy life."

## MAKING SENSE OF OUR SENSATIONS

What do "awfulizing," "I-can't-stand-it–itis" and "damnation," all have in common, beside the fact that they all lead to negative Cs or consequences? They all distort and exaggerate reality. And a great many negative beliefs, Ellis believes, are based on similarly incorrect, even irrational, premises. Obviously, the doctor's belief that Mary could not go home, and Paul's acceptance of that belief, *distorted* the reality that the family *could* care for Mary at home. And so does Eleanor's first reaction to her father's remark distort reality. Clearly, he did not intend to comment on breast cancer but to express his love for his wife and granddaughter.

Indeed, Eleanor's fear and dismay arose out of the distortion she imposed on his words, not on anything in the words themselves. According to rational emotive therapy, *irrational beliefs (iBs) lead to self-defeating ideas, feelings, and behaviors that bring on distress.*[1,2] Had Eleanor taken an *undistorted,* rational view of her father's comment, it would have caused her no distress. According to Ellis, *rational beliefs (rBs) lead to self-helping behaviors and limit distressing emotions, thoughts, and actions.*[1,2] Clearly, this was true for Laura. Instead of accepting the doctor's unfounded belief, she investigated the reality of caring for Mary at home. Then she was able to put together a realistic plan based on the real situation.

When Eleanor heard her father, on the other hand, she had an immediate, unconscious reaction that RET terms jumping to conclusions and negative *non sequitur* (Latin for "an action that does not follow"). She took a statement about physical appearance and automatically jumped to the illogical and inaccurate conclusion that this might imply a tendency toward breast cancer. Although similar appearance clearly indicates similar genetics, it does not constitute evidence that the genes related to breast cancer were also transmitted. Holly obviously shares some genes with her grandmother, but just as obviously, she does not share many more.

To shortcircuit the process that leads to distress, Eleanor could consciously work through this distortion and substitute for her automatic, irrational response a rational one that would not upset her. In his book *Feeling Good*, David Burns presents a specific method of doing this, called the "triple column" technique. It builds on Ellis's insight that we can substitute objective, rational thoughts for the irrational, negative thinking that can automatically flood our minds.[3]

The three-column technique is a method of analyzing your Bs—your beliefs, or what Burns calls your automatic thoughts, the ideas that first come into your head when you react to an activating event. The technique literally starts when you draw two lines on a sheet of paper (see figure.) Label the first one "automatic thought." Here you write down a thought that is negative and makes you feel uncomfortable. Next, label the middle column "cognitive distortion." Here you will indicate any errors in rational thinking that you can detect in your automatic thought. Finally, label the third column "rational response." Here you record a more rational interpretation of the event.

## "THREE-COLUMN" TECHNIQUE

| AUTOMATIC THOUGHT | COGNITIVE DISTORTION | RATIONAL RESPONSE |
|---|---|---|
| 1. I could have cancer and he doesn't care. | 1. Mind reading 2. Overgeneralization | 1. He doesn't know as much about cancer as I do. He may not realize how serious a biopsy can be. 2. He could be preoccupied with problems at work and not realize how worried I feel. 3. Maybe he's scared too and is handling his fear by avoiding the situation. |
| 2. He doesn't really love me and never has. | 1. Overgeneralization 2. All-or-nothing thinking | 1. Tom has been a loving husband for years. 2. If he knew how I felt, he'd care very much. Just because we haven't discussed my feelings about the biopsy doesn't mean he's stopped loving me. |

To show how this technique works, let's consider what happened when Ginnie's breast lump needed a biopsy. She felt that her husband, Tom, was preoccupied with himself, disinterested and unsupportive. Her automatic thought: "Here I could have cancer and he doesn't care. He doesn't really love me and never has." The feeling of being abandoned by the one she most depends on for support could easily plunge Ginnie into despair. But on calm consideration she can identify three examples of irrational thinking: First, she assumes without asking (mind reading) that he doesn't care; second, she feels that unless he shows total devotion he can't feel real love (all-or-nothing thinking); and finally, she generalizes by concluding that he never really loved her.

Now Ginnie can generate and test some alternatives. First there's "Perhaps Tom's preoccupied at work. I should tell him how scared I feel and that I need his attention." Then she thinks, "Maybe he's scared and is avoiding thinking about it."

Both possibilities require Ginnie to talk directly with Tom, express her feelings and needs, and request his support. Tom said "I'm so sorry. I had no idea you were so upset. You're usually so calm and in control of this breast business. I'm afraid I've been to focused on work, but obviously that's not nearly as important as what you're going through. Do you want to talk about it now? I was planning all along to go with you when you have the biopsy."

So Ginnie, through the three-column technique, discards a thought that would have distressed her and replaces it with another one that adds to her confidence: "Tom loves me and will support me through this trouble."

Her initial distress arose from automatic thinking in response to Tom's preoccupied manner, not from any objective merit that her thought may have. Once she realizes this, she can reject the irrational basis for her fears and concentrate instead on getting through the ordeal of biopsy.

Our detailed analysis of a small incident in Ginnie's life reveals a mechanism that, multiplied many times throughout each day, can cause a good deal of distress. We've identified a technique that effectively counters it. Applying this method in her daily life, every time she has a destructive automatic thought, Eleanor could greatly reduce her level of fear and anxiety.

If you still suspect that the techniques based on RET are

nothing more than simplistic "happy talk," we assure you that they are a great deal more. A large body of research has demonstrated that these methods can effectively impose discipline on our thinking and break the habits of thought that lead to unnecessary suffering. These methods do not imply that *all* distress is avoidable. Clearly, every life contains its share of trauma, pain, loss, and grief. But these methods, which have been proven over years of successful application in psychotherapy, can help to keep us from suffering needlessly and to recover from adversity less painfully.

## MENDING BAD HABITS

But can we really put this technique into daily practice? Can we change our habitual ways of thinking?

One reason that automatic thoughts have such a hold on our emotions is precisely because they're automatic. We're not any more aware of them than we are of most other automatic functions of our body, such as our breathing, heart rate, and blood pressure. Our eyes, for example, see automatically. But suppose you were wearing yellow-tinted lenses but didn't know it. Everything you saw would look yellower than it was, and you would think that the world's jaundiced appearance was natural, not the result of your lenses. Automatic thinking works in just the same way. Looking through the lens of anxiety about breast cancer, neither Eleanor nor Ginnie realizes that she's seeing a distorted reality.

If, however, we became aware of the tinted specs, we could either take them off, or, if that were not possible, we could consciously correct for the distortion they cause. In just the same way, *overcoming disturbing automatic thinking requires that we first become aware of it so that we can counter it.*

In 1976, Dr. Aaron Beck, a psychiatrist, proposed a way: the method he calls "Daily Record of Dysfunctional

Thoughts" derives from his system of cognitive therapy, which builds on Ellis's RET.[4] It helps an individual become aware of her patterns of thinking in response to everyday events. This in turn lets her know when she should use the three-column technique to counter negative thoughts. Thus it builds practical understanding of the relationship between thoughts, emotions, and behaviors and forms a basis for changing destructive patterns.

The Daily Record method consists of keeping a special sort of diary for a number of days. Decide to carry a notebook or pad and pencil with you for a few days. When you start feeling depressed, anxious, worried, or unhappy in a particular situation, you should write down the answers to five questions.

1. Describe the situation. What was I doing or thinking when the feeling started?
2. What form did the uncomfortable feeling take (anger, depression, irritation, anxiety, etc.)? How bad did I feel (very depressed, slightly irritated, etc.)?
3. What automatic thoughts preceded my emotions? What was going through my mind when the bad feeling started?
4. Are the negative thoughts realistic? What arguments can I use to refute them? What are some rational responses to my automatic thoughts?
5. How do I feel after I have tried to refute the negative thoughts? Do I still believe my automatic thoughts?

To see how this method works, let's take an example replacing distorted, negative thoughts with more accurate ones. We'll watch Emily go through the exercise, expanding on a comment we heard her make some chapters back: that a man might not want to enter a relationship with her because of her high-risk status.

At a dinner at the home of friends, Emily meets Bill, an attractive single man who shares many of her interests. The attraction is mutual and a couple of days later he calls to ask her out. Right now, Emily is studying her closet, considering what she should wear for their date tomorrow evening. Is the black dress most appropriate for the theater, or should she wear the blue silk outfit or the gray suit? Which would he like best? She thinks back to the dinner when they met.

"Bill seems like a really nice guy," she says to herself. "He speaks intelligently and has a great sense of humor. He's also quite good-looking. Plus, he roomed with my good friend Mike before Mike's marriage. I think that vouches for his character. He really seems like the sort of guy I could get serious about."

Now, as she takes out the blue silk, she speculates on whether Bill might share her feelings. After a series of relationships that haven't worked out, she'd really like to marry. Bill seems like a better and better candidate.

"I wonder if he wants a serious relationship," she thinks. "I wonder if he'll want to get to know me better after tomorrow. I wonder if he'll want to become involved with someone like me."

And then, suddenly: "I wonder if he'll want to get involved with someone who has my family history of breast cancer." Now her heart drops and her happy mood evaporates. "Why should he—why should any man want to take on something like that if he doesn't have to? Why should he want to involve himself with someone who faces that high a risk? Why should he do that for someone he doesn't even know?"

Now her mind is racing. "He won't. Even if he's interested in me at first, he'd probably drop me when he found out. No, this relationship won't work out any better than any of the others. No man will want to take the risk of getting involved with someone with my family background. I'll never find someone to marry. I'll end up alone."

Emily's happy reverie is long gone, her hope and enthusiasm replaced by apprehension, sorrow, and self-pity.

Now that we've watched Emily work herself up (or down) to the verge of depression, let's watch her take action by filling out, question by question, her thought record for this incident.

1. *What was I doing when the bad feeling started?* Here she describes choosing the outfit and thinking about the date.
2. *What form did the feeling take?* She indicates that she feels quite bad, depressed, apprehensive, and alone.
3. *What was going through my mind when the bad feeling started?* Here she reaches the crux of the matter, her automatic thought: "No man will want to take the risk of getting involved with someone with my family background."
4. *Is this thought realistic? Can I refute it?* Here she analyzes her idea about men. Just how likely is it that a family history of breast cancer would weigh so heavily in someone's feelings? Would it, for example, have the same influence on her? Wouldn't she assume that everyone was probably at risk for some disease? If she knew, for example, that Bill came from a family with a tendency toward a certain cancer, would that be enough to convince her not to get involved with him, if everything else in the relationship seemed favorable?

   "Of course it wouldn't," Emily says. "Having a family history is no guarantee of getting the disease. And even if it were, it's no guarantee that you'd die from it. That wouldn't keep me from falling in love with someone. And no decent person would abandon someone they loved because she might get sick."

What's more, Bill is an old, close friend of Mike's, and therefore probably a person of good character. Is it likely that Mike would remain friends with someone who's fickle, who judges people on such a superficial basis?

"Of course not," Emily thinks. "I just have to stop blaming my family history for what goes wrong in my life."

5. *How do I feel after refuting the negative thoughts?* Here Emily considers the outcome of this exercise. "I feel much more hopeful about my chances with Bill. I'm really looking forward to our date tomorrow. He seemed like fun and I'm sure we'll have a good time."

If you consciously keep a thought record for one week, you'll begin to recognize patterns of automatic thinking that increase your own distress about your high-risk status. You may see that like many of the women in this book, you habitually think of the worst possibilities. Keeping the record will give you practice in consciously countering your negative beliefs, which will short-circuit the process leading to distress. After you've become adept at answering the questions, you'll be able to continue this same process automatically. You'll be well on your way to controlling the anxiety and distress connected with being at high risk.

## LEARNING TO RELAX

By now, we hope that you've begun to see the power of the tools at your disposal. We've shown effective methods to work with negative self-talk and to recognize the main pitfalls on the road to healthy adjustment to high-risk status. In addition to cognitive techniques, there's another approach to controlling anxiety that every high-risk woman should know: physical training that produces the "relaxation response." Medical researcher Dr. Herbert Benson gave this name to the combination of lowered heart rate, breathing rate, blood pressure, and muscle tension that accompanies a feeling of relaxation.[5] (You probably recognize a racing heart, tense muscles, and rapid breathing as outward signs of anxiety.) Along with these altered physiological states, he found, go altered mental ones: a significant drop in anxiety and an increase of control over your thoughts.

Ginnie, for example, accomplishes this quite effectively before her mammogram appointment, which she dreads. First, she deploys her cognitive resources to get her thinking under control. "Before I go to my appointment," she says, "I think of the thing that worries me most: that I wouldn't be able to cope if I got a bad result." Then she carefully marshals her ideas to refute this thought: "I picture the possibility that I got a bad result, and I discuss with my husband what I would do if that happened—who I would call, what I would say, everything that would happen. I make a careful plan. That gives me more confidence that I'll be able to cope."

And then she does something else. "Before I go to my appointment, I do my relaxation exercises."

The benefits of relaxation training are neither ephemeral nor theoretical, researchers have found. It has been shown to help control anxiety in stressful situations. It combines perfectly with our cognitive techniques to significantly increase a woman's control over distress.

So useful are relaxation training methods, in fact, and so attainable is the relaxation response that in 1981 Benson, Borysenko, and colleagues founded the Mind-Body Clinic of Harvard University to spread the word that individuals can do it themselves.[6] The clinic teaches muscle relaxation and cognitive therapy as means to help people experience physical calm while learning physiological control over their reactions to the circumstances in their lives.

And just as you can deflect negative thinking, *you can also learn relaxation techniques that will help you control stress and anxiety.* If you practice them daily—several only take a few minutes—you will find the general level of tension in your life diminishing. And once you've become adept at them, you can, like Ginnie, consciously use them any time you want to conquer the anxiety that stands in the way of your early detection program or your general peace of mind. In the changing room before your mammogram, in the waiting room while waiting for the result, in your own home before your BSE, anytime, anywhere that anxiety arises, you'll be able to calm yourself. And that will give you the serenity needed to counter irrational thoughts. Together, these techniques form a unified strategy for making sure that you and not your fears control your mind and feelings.

We're going to detail two methods of relaxing that you can easily learn and practice completely on your own, starting today. They are progressive muscle relaxation, which tenses and then relaxes the body's various muscle groups, and three-dimensional breathing, which focuses attention on full and complete breathing through various parts of the body.

These exercises are most effective when practiced daily in a quiet environment. Practicing each day for approximately ten minutes will enable you to relax in anxiety-producing situations. You'll learn to modify the activity of your nervous system and lower your heart rate, blood pressure, and breathing rate. You'll experience how your mental state affects your bodily process and how your body in turn influences your thinking. Thus, when you feel the old anxiety and distress begin to overtake you, you'll have resources that you can mobilize to defeat it.

## MUSCLE RELAXATION

Until now we've discussed anxiety and tension as the emotional results of traumatic experiences and destructive thoughts. But they're far more than mere states of mind. Tension has a physical form, which affects the muscles and prevents you from relaxing either mentally or physically. By systematically relaxing your muscles, however, you can release that harmful grip. The simple exercise of progressive muscle relaxation, originally developed by Dr. Edmund Jacobson in the 1960s, teaches you how to do that.[7] Using it only a few minutes a day, you can learn to recognize the difference between muscle tension and muscle relaxation. Then you will be able to relax your muscles at will, relaxing your mind at the same time.

Seated comfortably, you'll sequentially tense and release major groups of muscles. Be sure to hold your breath while tensing and then exhale, breathing fully, while relaxing. We start at the bottom and work up.

1. First, while holding your breath, point your toes. Now point them harder. Let go of the tension and take a deep breath. Then repeat.

Now flex your toes and feet back. Pull up hard. Harder! Let go and breathe. Repeat.

2. Straighten your knees and press your thighs down into the chair. Press hard. Harder and straighter! Let go and breathe fully. Repeat.

3. Push your chest forward until your back is very arched. Lift more and push. Harder! Let go and breathe. Repeat.

4. Push your abdominal muscles out. Press out as hard as you can. Make your abdominals very tense. Let go and breathe. Repeat.

5. Press your palms together in front of your chest, mak-

ing your chest, arms, and hands very tight. Press harder. Let go and relax. Repeat.

6. Imagine you are holding back the reins on a runaway horse. Make fists and pull them in tightly to your chest. Pull your chin toward your chest. Pull tighter. Tighter! Let go and breathe. Then repeat.

7. Shrug your shoulders up around your ears. Pull them up tightly. Tighter! Let go and breathe. Repeat.

8. Scrunch your face up around your nose. Squeeze hard; you'll see colors as your eyes shut tightly. Harder! Let go and breathe.

9. Open up your face by opening eyes wide and sticking out your tongue. Open as wide as you can. Wider. Let go and breathe.

10. Now that you've tightened and released many major muscle groups, let yourself feel the relaxation throughout your body. Close your eyes, turn in toward yourself and relax. Relax your feet and lower legs. Let go in your knees and thighs. Relax your whole legs. Relax your hips and buttocks. Let go in the abdomen. Take a deep breath. Relax your chest and ribs and breathe deeply. Let go in your arms and hands. Let them rest at your sides. Relax your shoulders. Let your neck go loose and roll it around. Relax your face, relax your eyes. Feel your scalp relax. Take a deep breath and try to carry the relaxation you feel throughout the day.

## AN AIR OF RELAXATION

Ever notice how, when you feel stressed and anxious, your breathing becomes rapid and shallow? Or how deep, slow breathing goes with a feeling of serenity? Breathing can definitely affect our state of mind. But of all the natural, involuntary processes that affect our physiology, it's the easiest to bring under conscious control. In the next exercise, we make use of the fact that the brain's center closely communicates with its arousal center.

Calm, relaxed complete breathing, the kind that banishes tension and anxiety, is easy to learn. Three-dimensional breathing, a process developed by Dr. Renee Royak-Schaler, helps lower physical, mental, and emotional arousal and enhances your feeling of well-being.

1. Sitting in a chair or on the floor, place your hands on your upper chest, your fingers to your collarbone. Take a deep breath and exhale fully. Now, counting very slowly to five, inhale into your upper chest so that your collarbone lifts your hands. Now, to the count of five, slowly exhale. Repeat twice more.

2. Place your hands on your ribs at your sides. Imagine that this part of your body is like a butterfly's wings or a fish's gills. Take a deep breath and exhale fully. Now breathe into the rib cage to the slow count of five, feeling the muscles between your ribs expand. Now exhale, counting slowly to five, feeling the muscles contract. Do this three times.

3. Place your hands on your lower abdomen or pelvis. Imagine this part of your body to be a bowl that can be filled or emptied. Take a deep breath and exhale fully. Now inhale into the lower abdomen to the slow count of five, feeling the expansion in your hips. Now exhale, counting slowly to five, feeling your hips contract.

4. Let your hands rest at your sides. Take a deep breath and exhale fully. Now, while counting to five, breathe in turn into all three areas, upper chest, rib cage, and lower abdomen. Now exhale slowly. Do this three times.

At the end of this exercise, notice how easily you're breathing and how relaxed you feel.

## IN SUMMARY

We've given you many techniques, both cognitive and physical, that are proven to reduce anxiety and stress and put you back in control of your thoughts and feelings. Now it's time to try them out and see how they work for you. *It's important to give them a fair trial, using each daily for a few weeks so that results can accumulate.* Stay with them and they will become powerful weapons in your campaign against the negative emotional consequences of high-risk status.

Then, whenever you need to, you can alter negative thinking and relax yourself at will. When the time comes for your BSE and you feel yourself tense up, or while taking off your blouse for your mammogram you feel your heart begin to race, or if a friend's or relative's symptoms stir up the old anguish, you'll know what to do.

The greatest benefits of the relaxation techniques accrue to people who practice the exercises daily. With practice, the relaxation response becomes more and more automatic and easier to bring on at will.

The cognitive techniques of countering negative thinking and the physical techniques of bringing on the relaxation response will enable you to control distress and anxiety; in the last chapter we called this cognitive control.

The next chapter and the Afterword present the specific skills of behavioral control; these techniques of early detection, exercise, and good diet safeguard your health.

# 12

❦

# *Early Detection, Diet, and Exercise*

THERE'S ALWAYS something you can do," Martha says. She's right. And now that we've given you the tools for more effective emotion-focused coping, this chapter is going to equip you for effective problem-focused coping. Specifically, we will present what you need to know to carry out your program of regular mammograms, breast self-exams, and clinical breast exams, plus proper diet and exercise. Together, these add up to the best protection medical science offers a high-risk woman today. (All women, in fact, regardless of their risk status, would benefit from following this program.) Separately, none of these techniques is difficult to learn. Together—and in conjunction with the techniques presented in the preceding three chapters—they constitute a consistent approach that has helped high-risk women overcome danger and distress and enrich their lives.

If you use these techniques, they will definitely help you defeat anxiety, manage early detection, and develop a feeling of strength and competence in many areas of your life. They may also lower your chances of getting breast cancer, though the evidence here is more problematic.

By practicing the skills in this chapter, you'll alter both the behaviors and the feelings surrounding high-risk status. As you experience that you can change this aspect of your life, you'll gain an increased sense of mastery in other areas, too. This feeling of competence, experience shows, spreads beyond the realm of health behaviors to enrich all aspects of your life.

## EARLY DETECTION

It's time to speak frankly about the trio of vital exams that together constitute early detection. If you find them frightening or distasteful, you're not alone.

"Every time I examine myself, I'm sure I'll find a lump," says Lee.

"I try to remember to do it, but every month I'm still scared," says Anne.

"I'm just too terrified to examine myself," says Abby.

Almost nobody, in fact, not even the minority of women who practice breast self-examination regularly, likes to do it. And the same goes for mammography and clinical breast exam. Almost everyone would prefer to let all three of them slide. They're scary. They're a nuisance. They can be uncomfortable. Some people find them embarrassing.

And, perhaps most importantly, every four weeks they make us face the possibility of cancer. Month after month they stir up the fear and anxiety that all of us try so hard—and many of us actually manage—to bury most of the time. So if you share this distaste for any of the early detection techniques, you're not alone. You're not only normal, you're in the overwhelming majority.

But even as we acknowledge all the difficulties, there's something about these techniques that we think outweighs everything else—something we hope we can convince you of, too. *Without any doubt, these techniques save lives. Practiced properly and regularly, they are our single best means of protecting our health. The most important thing a high-risk woman can do is overcome the very natural resistance that she feels toward these practices so that she can do them regularly.*

Consider this. In 1943, the year that G. N. Papanicolaou and H. F. Traut first introduced the Pap smear, about the same numbers of Americans died of uterine and breast cancer—about 30,000 each, in a population much smaller than today's. This year, while breast cancer will take over 44,000 lives, uterine cancer will take approximately 10,000—thanks almost exclusively to the habit of the annual Pap.[1] Before the Pap, there was no reliable way to detect uterine cancer early enough to save lives. After it, millions of women who would certainly have died of cancer went on to live long, healthy lives. The death rate from uterine cancer has dropped over 70 percent in forty years. It would fall even farther—much closer to the 0 percent that is theoretically possible—if every woman took full advantage of the immensely powerful but very simple Pap test.

BSE, mammogram, and clinical breast exam could do something similar for breast cancer, if we used them as intensively. That possibility makes us perhaps the most fortunate generation of women who have ever lived, because we have the most powerful defenses against breast cancer that have ever existed. If every woman viewed her breast care as she does her Pap smear, if everyone took advantage of the power we have to detect breast cancer early, that toll would drop rapidly, too.

## TWO WAYS OF SEEING

BSE is the procedure that most women like least, because we have to do it ourselves, and often do it when we're alone. But it can save your life. In an English study, *women who had received instruction in breast self-exam had, after thirteen years, better survival than those who had not. And when the instructed women did develop cancer, the tumors were detected smaller, earlier, and with less spread.*[2]

But BSE and the mammogram don't substitute for one another. Eleanor, for example, knows a woman who "saved her own life" by having a mammogram after two doctors assured her that the lump she felt was "probably OK." It wasn't, but only the combination of the hand and machine made diagnosis certain. *To be fully protected, you need to use both.*

In doing BSE, fear can be a very real factor. Many of us, alone in the shower or lying on the bed, have found lumps. Many of us felt that sudden, sinking terror.

That may be what's holding you back from doing your monthly BSE, the memory or the fear of such an incident. But if so, consider this: *The great majority of lumps that women find are not cancerous. In fact, they're not even dangerous.* There are, in fact, four different kinds of lumps you don't have to worry about.

- The first are cysts, nothing more than harmless sacs of tissue filled with fluid that your doctor can easily drain by aspiration. Breast cysts are usually spherical, movable, and soft. They may be painful or not, and their symptoms may be most noticeable before a menstrual period. A woman may have one or multiple cysts.
- The second are fibroadenomas, which are solid, benign tumors composed of fibrous and glandular tissues. They

are painless, movable, and rubbery, and can occur in multiples. They can easily be seen on a mammogram, but can be distinguished from breast cancer only by biopsy after they are removed.

- The third are intraductal papillomas, small wartlike growths in the mammary duct lining near the nipple. They typically involve bleeding from the nipple, and are treated by surgically removing the involved duct.
- The fourth are lumps from areas of infection or abscess, called mastitis. This condition is usually caused by bacteria and is found in women who are breast feeding. It is treated with antibiotics.[3]

"My breasts are full of lumps," says Abby, explaining why she doesn't do regular BSE. But everyone's breasts feel lumpy at least part of the time. When you do BSE, you're not really examining yourself for lumps; you're looking for *new* lumps, for *changes* in your tissue that indicate changes in your cells.

"Doing your monthly exam will let you learn what's normal for you," Sheila says. It will take some time to become familiar with the feel of your breasts. As you do, you will gain more confidence about doing the exam.

## DOING BSE

A self-exam only takes a few minutes. It's important, though, that you do it at the same time each month. As long as you have your periods, your breasts change from week to week, become more or less swollen, more or less lumpy. It's best, therefore, to pick a time when they're least likely to be swollen or extra lumpy, generally about a week to ten days after the beginning of your period. If your periods have stopped, then pick a day of the month—the first or fifteenth or whatever—to do your exam every time. The following method of breast self-exam is recommended by the American Cancer Society.

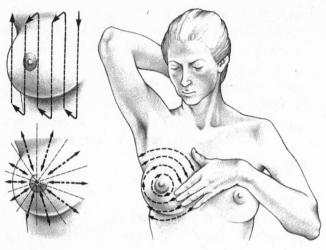

Start your self-exam by standing undressed before a mirror.

1. Look closely at each breast, checking for any visible lumps, indentations, wrinkling, or changes in texture. Also note if there's been any change in the nipple.
2. Then raise both arms and check for swollen or dimpled areas.
3. Next, clasp your hands behind your head, your elbows apart, still watching for changes.
4. Now, put your hands on your hips and bring your elbows and shoulders forward, eyes still on the mirror.
5. Next, still standing, with your left hand, carefully feel your entire right breast. You might want to do this in the shower. To make sure you cover all parts of the breast, move your hand according to any one of three patterns:

- Vertical stripes. Imagine that your breast is tattooed with stripes running from your shoulder to your abdomen. Move your hand carefully along each strip, starting at the top of the innermost strip and working down. When you reach the bottom of the first strip, work your way up the second. Continue, working from top to bottom, until you have covered the entire breast.
- Spiral. Imagine that your breast is tattooed with a spiral that starts at the top and circles around and around, homing in on the nipple. Starting at the top, move your hand carefully along the curve until you reach the nipple.
- Wedges. Imagine that your breast is a pie, divided into six or eight wedges. Starting at the outside edge, move your hand back and forth until you cover an entire wedge, then go on to the adjacent wedge, and so on until you do them all.

Which of these systems you choose makes no difference. The important thing is that *you examine your breast completely*.

6. Next, squeeze your nipple and note if you see any discharge.
7. Then, use the right hand to examine the left breast thoroughly in the same manner. It is common to notice differences in appearance, form, and texture between your breasts. They are not necessarily mirror images of one another.
8. Finally, lie on your bed or couch. With a towel or pillow under the left shoulder, use the right hand to repeat the stripe, spiral, or wedge pattern. Then move your towel or pillow to the other side and repeat the procedure.[4] You can contact your local chapter of ACS or call 1-800-ACS-2345 to obtain a copy of the pam-

phlet "Special Touch," which contains these breast self-exam guidelines.

*Notify your doctor immediately if you find any new lump or thickening or if you have any discharge (and you're not breast feeding).*

Finding something, of course, may be very distressing, awakening fear and frightening memories. But should it happen, *remember that the great majority of lumps are harmless.* This is the time to use your cognitive and relaxation skills to help cope with your fear. Keep in mind that lumps that feel round or that move about are less likely to be cancerous. *But don't try to diagnose breast irregularities yourself. This is the business of a trained and experienced expert: your doctor.*

Because the key to successful BSE is finding the lump that's abnormal for you, a good way to get started is to have your doctor or a nurse at your breast center show you how it's done and help you get the feel of "normal" and "abnormal" lumps. Most centers have lifelike model breasts that give you hands-on training.


## THE MAMMOGRAM

You should have a mammogram taken as often as your medical adviser thinks necessary. As we noted in Chapter 6, this may vary according to your age, your level of risk, and your state of breast health. It will certainly be once a year or more often. This X-ray picture of your breast will show irregularities too small to be felt by hand. It also records the status of your breast at a given moment and permits comparisons over time that can show changes. All women should have their first, or baseline, mammogram between ages thirty-five and forty. Many high-risk women should start sooner. If you haven't yet started having mammograms, you should discuss the precise timing with your doctor.

Many women find the actual process of mammography a bit uncomfortable. The key to an accurate picture—and therefore to an accurate reading—is adequate compression. Especially if your breasts are large, therefore, the technician may have to use a fair amount of pressure. But remember, the exposure itself takes only seconds and the machine releases your tissue instantly.

Discuss with your doctor or breast center the best place in your community to have your mammograms done. It's important that a skilled technician take the picture and that a fully trained and experienced radiologist—preferably one who does many such readings—interprets it. Many high-risk women feel added confidence at a hospital breast center, which is likely to have doctors who specialize in breast disease.

## THE MEDICAL BREAST EXAM

Your doctor or a breast center nurse will also perform your clinical breast exam—a manual examination similar to BSE. This includes visual inspection, looking for changes in shape or size, or dimpling of the skin, followed by a thorough manual inspection of the breasts, chest, and armpit. Some high-risk women feel that this is where breast centers really shine, because their personnel do enough clinical breast exams to be truly expert. "They're so thorough," Sheila says, laughing, "that when you leave, your breasts are sore." Again, the precise timing depends on your individual case. Some people, like Abby, go every three months; some, like Anne, every six months.

\*    \*    \*

Undertaking these three steps means doing the most important things to safeguard your health. It also means that you have taken charge of an uncertain situation. You, like millions of other women, *can* practice early detection properly and effectively. *The commitment to do so is a mark of your determination to do all you can to safeguard your health.*

## EATING RIGHT

The next element of our strategy for healthy living is a low-fat diet. The scientific debate on fat and breast cancer goes on, but evidence continues to pile up.

High-fat diets clearly stimulate mammary tumors in rats. When female rats ate a diet low in fat or low in calories regardless of fat level, or when they could exercise at will, they had fewer mammary tumors, according to Dr. Leonard Cohen and colleagues at the American Health Foundation.[5] So did rats fed high fiber along with high fat. The breast cancer rate of Finnish women—half that of Americans—first suggested this possibility to Cohen's group. In Finland, people eat as much fat as Americans but a great deal more fiber, and they have a breast cancer incidence far lower than either Americans or their north European neighbors.[6] Laboratory animal studies are consistent with studies of cancer incidence in human populations in suggesting that fat intake correlates with breast cancer, particularly after menopause. And tumor incidence correlates with body weight and daily caloric intake.

Scientists believe that the amount of estrogen circulating in a woman's blood influences her likelihood of developing the disease. Some theorize that dietary fiber may reduce that level, although Cohen's group didn't find that result. Still, American women who eat a lot of fat and little fiber have much higher circulating estrogen levels than Asian women who eat half as much fat and much more fiber. A number of experiments that tinkered with American women's diets, like the Women's Health Trial and the work of David Rose and Andrea Boyar, have found that reducing fat from 38 percent to 20 percent of calories significantly lowered serum estrogen levels. Adding wheat bran to a high-fat diet has had a similar result.[7]

So, although the connection is not yet definitive, we believe that *every high-risk woman should actively reduce the level of fat in her diet. And a number of studies have shown that American women can lower their fat intake if they wish.* It is neither complicated nor mysterious. It merely takes planning and determination.

The American Health Foundation's Food Plan presents a practical, useful approach, based on three Standards to Live By:[8]

• Reducing total fats to 25 percent of calories. On average, we Americans now get 37 percent of our daily calories from red meat, milk products, fried foods, and other high-fat dishes. Because each gram of fat contains nine calories, a daily diet of 2,000 calories of which 37 percent are fat contains eighty-two grams of fat. A 2,000-calorie diet containing 25 percent fat would have only fifty-six grams of fat. It's not hard to calculate the percentage of the calories in a food that comes from fat. You simply need to know the nutritional composition of the food, either from a package label or from a book that lists fat grams. To determine the percentage of fat, multiply the number of fat grams by nine and divide the result by the total number of calories. For example, a 200-calorie cookie that contains twelve grams of fat has 108 calories of fat and is 54 percent fat. That is to say: $12 \times 9 = 108$. $108 \div 200 = .54$, or 54%.

• Eating equal amounts of the three major types of fat—saturated, polyunsaturated, and monounsaturated. This means cutting back on meats and dairy products that contain satu-

204 A Program for Successful Living

rated fats, moderating vegetable oils from corn, safflower, and sesame seeds, which contain polyunsaturated fats, and switching to olive, peanut, and canola oils, which contain monounsaturated fats.

• Eating 25 grams of fiber each day, at least a third of it soluble. This means increasing dried beans, apples, oat and rice bran, citrus fruits, and carrots, which contain soluble fiber.

What does this mean in practice? It means paying attention to what you eat, asking yourself how you can reduce unnecessary fat and add extra fiber. Changing from a high-fat to a low-fat diet may mean changing your cooking habits. Like most people, for example, you probably use a fair amount of fat to grease pans. Try instead to cook with as little fat as possible; boil, bake, steam, braise, or stir-fry in broth. Try to avoid frying or sautéing. But when you must fry or sauté, use nonstick pans or a cooking spray instead of oil or butter. It means browning meat under the broiler instead of in fat.

Changing from a high-fat to a low-fat diet also means changing some of your choices in foods. For creamy, fatty foods such as salad dressings, sauces, and mayonnaise, you'll seek out lower-fat alternatives: lemon juice or fat-free dressings, for example; fat-free or low-fat mayonnaise, fat-free yogurt instead of or mixed with mayonnaise.

You'll also have to be careful when you get to the main course. Red meats represent a major part of most people's fat intake. Fish and skinless chicken offer tasty, versatile alternatives. But when you do eat red meats, choose lean cuts such as tenderloin or round in place of marbled or fatty cuts like chuck, brisket, and rib. Choose extra-lean ground beef, or make an even lower-fat mixture by combining extra-lean ground meat with low-fat ground turkey or fat-free tofu. Avoid fatty lunch meats, substituting white chicken or turkey meat. Avoid bacon and sausages.

At dessert time, at breakfast time, or for your coffee break, avoid fatty baked goods like cookies, layer cakes, pastries, or croissants. Choose instead such low-fat items as gingersnaps, angel food cake, English muffins, or bagels. Instead of potato or corn chips, choose popcorn (without butter) or pretzels.

Dairy foods are major contributors to most people's fat intake, and so wise choices in this area can make a real difference: skim milk instead of whole milk; low-fat cheeses instead of high-fat cheeses; yogurt instead of sour cream; evaporated skim milk instead of cream; whipped evaporated skim milk instead of whipped cream; frozen low-fat yogurt or sherbet instead of ice cream; two egg whites instead of an egg. Substitutions like these can add up to major reduction.

Adding fiber to the diet also means making careful choices. Whenever possible, use whole-grain breads, cereals, and baked goods in place of refined-flour, low-fiber ones. Use brown rice in place of white, bean or pea soups instead of clear broths or cream soups, mixed vegetable salads in place of plain lettuce. Choose whole fruits with skin instead of juices. A copy of the American Health Foundation's Food Plan, "Live Well the Low-Fat/High-Fiber Way," can be requested from the American Health Foundation, Publications, 1 Dana Road, Valhalla, NY 10595.

The American Cancer Society has also issued dietary recommendations to promote health and reduce rates of cancer. They suggest that you:

- Avoid obesity.
- Cut down on total fat intake.
- Eat more high-fiber foods such as whole-grain cereals, fruits, and vegetables.

- Include foods rich in vitamins A and C in your diet.
- Include cruciferous vegetables such as red and white cabbage, brussels sprouts, broccoli, kale, and cauliflower.
- Be moderate in alcohol consumption.
- Be moderate in consumption of salt-cured, smoked, and nitrite-cured foods.[9]

To judge how you're doing, take the American Cancer Society's Eating Smart Quiz, below.

## EATING SMART QUIZ

| OILS & FATS | | | POINTS |
|---|---|---|---|
| butter, margarine, shortening, mayonnaise, sour cream, lard, oil, salad dressing | I always add these foods in cooking and/or at the table. | 0 | ☐ |
| | I occasionally add these to foods in cooking and/or at the table. | 1 | |
| | I rarely add these to foods in cooking and/or at the table. | 2 | |
| | I eat fried foods 3 or more times a week. | 0 | ☐ |
| | I eat fried foods 1–2 times a week. | 1 | |
| | I rarely eat fried foods. | 2 | |

| DAIRY PRODUCTS | | | POINTS |
|---|---|---|---|
| | I drink whole milk. | 0 | |
| | I drink 1–2% fat-free milk | 1 | |
| | I seldom eat frozen desserts or ice cream. | 2 | |
| | I eat ice cream almost every day. | 0 | |
| | Instead of ice cream, I eat ice milk, low-fat frozen yogurt & sherbet. | 1 | |
| | I eat only fruit ices, seldom eat frozen dairy dessert. | 2 | |
| | I eat mostly high-fat cheese (jack, cheddar, colby, Swiss, cream). | 0 | |
| | I eat both low- and high-fat cheeses. | 1 | |
| | I eat mostly low-fat cheeses (pot, 2% cottage, skim milk mozzarella). | 2 | |

| SNACKS | | | POINTS |
|---|---|---|---|
| potato/corn chips, nuts, buttered popcorn, candy bars | I eat these every day. | 0 | |
| | I eat some occasionally. | 1 | |
| | I seldom or never eat these snacks. | 2 | |

| BAKED GOODS | | | |
|---|---|---|---|
| pies, cakes, cookies, sweet rolls, doughnuts | I eat them 5 or more times a week. | 0 | |
| | I eat them 2–4 times a week. | 1 | |
| | I seldom eat baked goods or eat only low-fat baked goods. | 2 | |

| POULTRY & FISH* | | POINTS |
|---|---|---|
| | I rarely eat these foods.  0 | |
| | I eat them 1–2 times a week.  1 | |
| | I eat them 3 or more times a week.  2 | |

| LOW-FAT MEATS* | | |
|---|---|---|
| extra lean hamburger, round steak, pork loin roast, tenderloin, chuck roast | I rarely eat these foods.  0 | |
| | I eat these foods occasionally.  1 | |
| | I eat mostly fat-trimmed red meats.  2 | |

| HIGH-FAT MEAT* | | |
|---|---|---|
| luncheon meats, bacon, hot dogs, sausage, steak, regular & lean ground beef | I eat these every day.  0 | |
| | I eat these foods occasionally.  1 | |
| | I rarely eat these foods.  2 | |

| CURED & SMOKED MEAT & FISH* | | |
|---|---|---|
| luncheon meats, hot dogs, bacon, ham & other smoked or pickled meats and fish | I eat these foods 4 or more times a week.  0 | |
| | I eat some 1–3 times a week.  1 | |
| | I seldom eat these foods.  2 | |

| LEGUMES | | |
|---|---|---|
| dried beans & peas: kidney, navy, lima, pinto, garbanzo, split-pea, lentil | I eat legumes less than once a week.  0 | |
| | I eat these foods 1–2 times a week.  1 | |
| | I eat them 3 or more times a week.  2 | |

*If you do not eat meat, fish or poultry, give yourself a 2 for each meat category.

## WHOLE GRAINS & CEREALS                                    POINTS

| whole grain breads, brown rice, pasta, whole grain cereals | I seldom eat such foods. | 0 | |
| | I eat them 2–3 times a day. | 1 | |
| | I eat them 4 or more times daily. | 2 | |

## VITAMIN C-RICH FRUITS & VEGETABLES

| citrus fruits and juices, green peppers, strawberries, tomatoes | I seldom eat them. | 0 | |
| | I eat them 3–5 times a week. | 1 | |
| | I eat them daily. | 2 | |

## DARK GREEN & DEEP YELLOW FRUITS & VEGETABLES*

| broccoli, green, carrots, peaches | I seldom eat them. | 0 | |
| | I eat them 3–5 times a week. | 1 | |
| | I eat them daily. | 2 | |

## VEGETABLES OF THE CABBAGE FAMILY

| broccoli, cabbage, brussels sprouts, cauliflower | I seldom eat them. | 0 | |
| | I eat them 1–2 times a week. | 1 | |
| | I eat them 3–4 times a week. | 2 | |

## ALCOHOL

| | I drink more than 2 oz. daily. | 0 | |
| | I drink alcohol every week but not daily. | 1 | |
| | I occasionally or never drink alcohol. | 2 | |

*Dark green and yellow fruits and vegetables contain beta carotene, which your body can turn into vitamin A and which helps protect you against certain types of cancer-causing substances.

PERSONAL WEIGHT

I'm more than 20 lbs. over my ideal weight.     0
I'm 10–20 lbs. over my ideal weight.     1
I am within 10 lbs. of my ideal weight.     2

Total Score

## How Do You Rate?

*0–12: A Warning Signal*
Your diet is too high in fat and too low in fiber-rich foods. It would be wise to assess your eating habits to see where you could make improvements.

*13–17: Not Bad! You're Partway There*
You still have a way to go. Pay special attention to our dietary suggestions, though, and you might find some new ways to improve your diet.

*18–36: Good For You! You're Eating Smart*
You should feel very good about yourself. You have been careful to limit your fats and eat a varied diet. Keep up the good habits and continue to look for ways to improve.

## EXERCISE

Now we arrive at the final element of our program. Regular aerobic exercise, the kind that raises your heart rate and oxygen intake, benefits high-risk women in four ways. As we saw in Chapter 6, it effectively reduces tension, anxiety, and depression while it enhances self-esteem and feelings of competence and control. As we saw in our discussion of Rose Frisch's work in Chapter 5, it appears to reduce the risk of uterine, ovarian, cervical, and breast cancer. And finally, it improves a person's general state of health and may contribute to a longer lifespan. A study of 10,224 men and 3,120 women done in the 1980s by the Institute for Aerobics Research, for example, found that physical fitness reduces the risk of dying of heart disease and cancer.[10] Over an eight-year period, individuals who did least well on a treadmill fitness test had death rates twice as high as those who exercised moderately. And surprisingly little effort—simply walking briskly for thirty to sixty minutes a day, for example—provides this protection. Regular exercise appears to slow the processes associated with aging, allowing women to maintain lean muscle tissue, reduce body fat, and remain physically active well into middle and older age.

We believe that every high-risk woman should undertake a program of regular aerobic exercise. The form of exercise you choose makes no difference; what matters is finding something you like and staying with it. The American College of Sports Medicine provides four useful guidelines for achieving fitness. First, pick an aerobic or endurance exercise such as walking, jogging, hiking, swimming, skating, bicycling, cross-country skiing, or aerobic dancing. Second, do the activity three to five times a week. Third, do it continuously for fifteen to sixty minutes, depending on its intensity. And finally, exercise intensely enough to raise your pulse to between 50 and 85 percent of your maximum heart rate, a figure you can calculate by subtracting your age from 220.[11]

An effective program doesn't require joining a health club, hiring a personal trainer, buying expensive equipment, or having athletic talent. Most people, regardless of their age or weight, can get all the benefits of exercise safely, cheaply, and conveniently simply by taking a regular walk, a form of aerobic exercise that doesn't stress the bones or joints as jogging and aerobic dancing do. And unlike the 60 percent of joggers who quit within three months, walkers tend to stick with their exercise regimes.[12]

Walking has comprehensive benefits that affect many

body systems. It improves the strength and efficiency of the heart and lungs, stimulates the circulation and helps lower blood pressure. As the heart becomes more efficient, it can pump more blood in each beat. Thus, heart rate slows, the number of red blood cells increase, blood and oxygen supplies to the tissues increase, and resting blood pressure falls. Walking also positively affects cholesterol and triglyceride levels. Lipoprotein molecules carry cholesterol in the blood; high-density lipoproteins (HDLs) pick up excess cholesterol and carry it to the liver for elimination. Low-density lipoproteins, on the other hand, stick to the walls of the coronary arteries and promote heart disease. Walking increases the HDLs and thus reduces your risk of heart disease.

Weight-bearing activities like walking also strengthen the bones, regardless of one's age, and may retard the osteoporosis that accompanies aging in many women. Walking uses most of the body's 660 muscles and 206 bones.[13] This gains in importance as we age and "use it or lose it" becomes the operative rule. A 1986 study of postmenopausal women, for example, found that levels of aerobic fitness relate to bone density in the spine and hip.[14]

Walking also improves the strength and flexibility of joints and muscles. As the legs tone, the other muscles, ligaments, tendons, and cartilage involved in bearing weight also strengthen. Regular walking builds weak abdominal and spinal muscles, improving posture and enhancing flexibility in the spine, hips, and legs, all of which help reduce back pain.

Regular exercise burns calories and helps regulate energy balance and body weight. A physically fit individual develops a more efficient metabolism that aids in weight control. Only an integrated program of exercise and diet leads to lifelong weight control.[15] Walking has been shown to increase muscle mass while helping to reduce body fat.

Regular exercise also enhances self-image and appearance.

It also reduces anxiety and depression by speeding the break-down of stress-related hormones and also appears to encourage the brain to produce more endorphins, compounds believed responsible for the feeling of well-being associated with exercise.[16] Mastering a form of exercise, be it brisk walking, jogging, aerobic dancing, or whatever, can build a woman's belief in her capability and competence; this new confidence often spreads to other spheres of life, enhancing her self-esteem. Conditioning exercises can also decrease uncomfortable premenstrual symptoms like breast tenderness, fluid retention, and depression.[17]

## Getting Started

To begin your walking program, we suggest you take the Rockport Fitness Walking Test, developed in 1984 at the Exercise Physiology Laboratory at the University of Massachusetts Medical School.[12] You'll need to find a flat, measured mile to walk, usually available at a high school track. If you decide to measure your own course, choose someplace where you can walk continuously without interruptions.

The test also requires you to take your own pulse. Simply place your pointer and middle fingers either on the inside of your wrist or over the carotid artery in your neck. The rhythmic beating of your blood will tell you when you've found the right place. Now, using a watch to time yourself, count the beats for fifteen seconds and multiply that number by four to get your pulse rate for an entire minute. First take a resting pulse, which means you must be relaxed and seated. Typically, this will be between fifty and ninety beats per minute.

Now you're ready for the test proper, involving three simple steps. First, walk the mile as fast as you can while maintaining a steady pace. Second, record your time to the second; most people can do a mile in ten to twenty minutes.

Finally, take and record your pulse immediately after the walk. Don't wait even a few seconds, as your heart begins to slow as soon as you stop walking.[12]

To determine your fitness level, consult the chart on page 215, looking at the box appropriate for your age. You'll find scales indicating your time in minutes and your heart rate. A forty-five-year-old walker who takes fifteen minutes and thirty seconds and ends with a heart rate of 130 beats per minute, for example, rates above average in fitness.

Once you know your fitness level, you can begin one of the walking programs suggested by the Rockport Walking Institute and *Walking* magazine. Those in poor or low condition can realistically begin by walking for twenty-five or thirty minutes five times a week at three miles per hour, covering 1¼ to 1½ miles each time. A person in below average condition can start with thirty to thirty-five minutes five times a week at three miles per hour, for 1½ to 1¾ miles. If you're in average condition, you can do thirty-five to forty minutes at 3 to 3.5 miles per hour, or 2 miles, five times each week. Those in excellent or high condition can do forty-five to fifty minutes at 4 to 4.5 miles per hour, or 3 to 4 miles, five times a week. As your fitness increases, gradually increase your distance, but only add a quarter mile every two weeks. By the end of the first month, you'll probably want to speed up your pace as well, by about ½ mile per hour. You get maximum cardiovascular benefit when you exercise continuously at your target heart rate, 60 to 80 percent of your maximum heart rate.

We suggest that you adequately warm up and stretch your muscles before beginning your fitness walk and that you spend a few minutes at the end of each session slowing down and cooling off before you stop your exercise. Although you can undertake a perfectly satisfactory walking program on your own, many people find that it adds to their enjoyment to join

# WHAT IS YOUR FITNESS LEVEL?

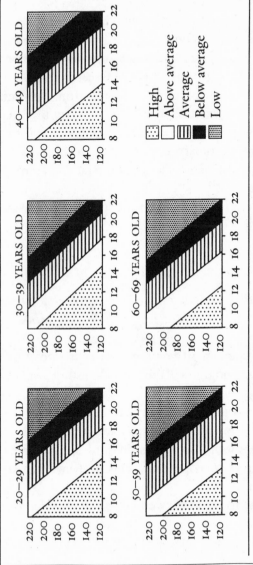

Legend:
- High
- Above average
- Average
- Below average
- Low

20—29 YEARS OLD

30—39 YEARS OLD

40—49 YEARS OLD

50—59 YEARS OLD

60—69 YEARS OLD

■ Vertical numbers indicate heartbeats per minute. ■ Horizontal numbers indicate time in minutes.

Reprinted by permission of the Rockport Walking Institute, 220 Donald J. Lynch Boulevard, Marlboro, MA 01752.

a group at a local Y or recreation department or begin a walking group with friends.

Although we don't yet know whether women who start regular exercise later in life enjoy the cancer-protective benefits of Harvard's college athletes, one suggestive finding comes from the rats. Two groups of female research animals were fed a diet deriving 40 percent of the calories from fat. One group had free access to exercise wheels, which they used regularly, and the other did not. The active group develop only one-third as many mammary tumors as the cage potatoes. And equally significantly, animals fed a high-fat diet seem naturally to choose exercise.[18]

A list of references that provide specific exercise programs appears in our Recommended Reading List.

## IN SUMMARY

Our strategy for living has taken a long section to present, but in practice you'll find it simple and straightforward:

- Take advantage of every means of early detection—regular mammograms, BSE, and clinical breast exams—to safeguard your health.
- Use the cognitive techniques in the previous two chapters to help control negative and irrational thinking.
- Use relaxation training techniques along with cognitive techniques to cope more effectively with anxiety and tension.
- Exercise for at least twenty-five minutes a minimum of three times a week.
- Eat a diet low in fat and high in fiber.

Each of these steps contributes to your health, your emotional well-being, and your sense of control over your life.

Together they will brighten your outlook and enrich your life.

Now you have the skills and knowledge you need to maximize your well-being as a high-risk woman. If you practice the methods of early detection, diet, and exercise, you can rest assured that you are doing all that is currently possible to protect your health. If you practice the cognitive and relaxation techniques, you will overcome anxiety, depression, and fear, the major obstacles to good monitoring and causes of much of the distress that high-risk women feel.

The rest is up to you. You now have major resources that can help you take control of your life. We hope that they will bring you the hope, optimism, and well-being that they have brought to many others.

# Afterword: Realistic Responsibility

❦

"CANCER OR no cancer, life's too short," Martha says. "You might as well enjoy it."

Martha's credo encapsulates what we've been trying to convey throughout this book. Life is for living. The challenge facing a high-risk woman is the same as that facing every human being; to live each day as richly, as satisfyingly, as positively as possible; to achieve the purposes and fulfill the potentials that give one's life meaning. But if a family legacy of breast cancer casts a special shadow over your days, you may find yourself dissipating your energies in anxiety, guilt, denial, or fear, rather than putting them toward accomplishing your broader and more valuable aims.

Only you can determine the goals you ought to pursue. Only you can evaluate your efforts to reach them. But the experiences of many high-risk women have led us to the methods suggested in this book. We believe that they will help free your mind from doubt and despair and empower you to work toward the purposes of your own choosing.

As things now stand, regretfully, neither we nor anyone else—regardless of what they claim—can guarantee that you may not someday face a diagnosis of breast cancer. (However, the odds of this happening to you are probably less than you're used to thinking. Furthermore, all women, not just high-risk women, face this danger to a greater or lesser extent.) Perhaps, with continued research, the day may come when that promise can honestly be made.

But even now, even with today's imperfect understanding, we can confidently give you this assurance: You already have the power to live your life fully regardless of what the future brings. You can make today and every day that is your portion into an opportunity for fulfilling your own goals.

*The key is realistic responsibility.* Please take note of this phrase. We've chosen these two words with care: *realistic* because an appreciation of your objective circumstances underlies all mature behavior; *responsibility* because the willingness to take charge of how you react to those circumstances will maximize both your emotional and your physical well-being.

*Taking realistic responsibility for your life means embracing the obligation—to yourself and to those who love you—to do all in your power to preserve your health.* It means acknowledging your ability both to alter your lifestyle and to affect your emotional reactions. It means accepting the need to stay informed about the factors affecting women like yourself. *But it does not mean accepting the blame for outcomes beyond your control.* It does not mean holding yourself accountable if, despite your best efforts, things do not turn out the way you want them to. It does not mean demanding that you be perfect.

Both scholarly research and a large popular literature discuss the correlation among behaviors, attitudes, and health outcomes experienced by cancer patients. It does appear, for example, that women who display "fighting spirit" may survive longer than those who show passive resignation.

But does this mean that individuals are "responsible" for their health outcome in the sense of having caused it? Do "unsuccessful" patients bear the blame for their "failure" to "conquer" cancer? Absolutely not, despite what some bestselling books may suggest. *The association between attitude and outcome is nothing more than a finding that two things often occur together.* Only in very rare cases can science now assign a specific cause to any particular cancer. A few cancers, for example, arise from known genes. Some cancer victims—workers at the Chernobyl plant who later died of leukemia, for example—have had massive exposures to known carcinogens.

But few people's lives contain such obvious patterns; if the factors causing breast cancers, for example, were so clear, scientists could pinpoint who will develop the disease. For now, and for the foreseeable future, they cannot. Therefore, any discussion of prevention now contains a sizable portion of guesswork. Following our strategy for daily living will maximize your chances of good health; it cannot guarantee them.

Therefore, *blaming either yourself for any inability to "prevent" cancer or your relatives for "causing" your risk status is not realistic.* Rather, it is unfair and punitive, the worst kind of irrational negative self-talk. No one can be held to account for what is not humanly possible. "Blaming the victim" does not represent true responsibility but rather its opposite. It is a technique that frightened people use to assure themselves of their own safety, a way of separating themselves from the possibility of bad fortune and from the uncertainty and ambiguity inherent in the human condition. By responsibility, we do not mean blame. Rather, we mean the understanding that no one but you can take charge of your own life.

Martha, for example, believes that her fate is ultimately beyond human control. "It's out of our hands," she says, but adds in the same breath, "I believe there's always something you can do." We hope that you, too, will take from this book a similar attitude of balance and determination. Martha asserts that she does not hold ultimate power, but still she strives to make the best use of the power she knows she has. She seeks out the highest quality medical care. She keeps herself informed. She cultivates healthy habits and a positive attitude. She exemplifies the approach that we believe offers high-risk women the best chance of a satisfying life: *Do everything you can, but realize that you can't do everything.*

## SPEAKING OUT

As we've seen many times in these pages, high-risk status is an extremely personal issue. Until now, it has almost always been played out within the boundaries of personal life. Even those celebrities—Betty Ford, Julia Child, Gloria Steinem, and others—who have gone public with their experiences and concerns have done so in the context of personal behavior, primarily by encouraging everyone to get regular screening.

But action can go beyond the personal. As the feminist movement pointed out two decades ago, "The personal is political." Personal experience exists within a framework of power relationships. And, across the country, women are waking up to the fact that our common health issues are more than the personal concerns of individuals. They are political issues that involve both the nation's spending priorities and the futures of millions of citizens of both sexes and all ages.

AIDS activists have shown the way in transforming a personal health concern into a national political priority. Their relentless campaign for attention and action has achieved big successes, even if much remains to be done. Thanks in large measure to their efforts, for example, the rules governing testing of certain drugs have been changed, making experimental treatments more available to sick people. And perhaps even more importantly, the federal government has for a number of years spent three-quarters of a *billion* dollars a year on AIDS research. Each year, by contrast, the government spends $70 million on breast cancer research, which *annually* kills two-thirds as many Americans as have died of AIDS up to now.

This shows the impact that concerted political action can produce.

The time is overdue for women to work together to transform our numbers and our anxieties about breast cancer into increased research and services. As we hope this book has helped empower you to take responsibility for your own health, we also hope that it will encourage you to begin thinking in terms of empowering yourself politically as well. We hope that you will begin using your power as a citizen to help improve the health of all women everywhere. Only more research will show us how to prevent breast cancer. And only more pressure from voters will produce the dollars needed to do that research. Our elected representatives will act in our behalf if they know that women's health issues are important to us.

The health concerns of women have not received attention from researchers equal to that given the health concerns of men. Over recent decades, for example, major funding has gone to long-term studies of heart disease, a major killer of both men and women, but one thought of primarily as a man's disease. And for many years, heart research essentially ignored women.

*It's time for the diseases that threaten the majority of our population—females—to get the attention they—and we—deserve. The concerted political power of women can make this happen. We owe it to our daughters and to ourselves to exercise this power.*

In fact, because of increased scrutiny by female public officials, things have already begun to change for the better and the health needs of women have begun to move onto the agendas of both scientists and legislators. In September 1990, the National Institutes of Health established a new Office of Research on Women's Health, charged with assuring that diseases that predominantly affect women—such as breast cancer—receive their fair share of attention from researchers. But the overall health of women in this country will only improve when all women have access to adequate preventive care. We have assumed throughout this book that our readers have the means or the insurance to obtain high-quality mammography and clinical services as often as their doctors deem it advisable.

For large numbers of women in this country, though, doubtlessly including some readers of these words, this assumption is false. Whether a high-risk woman has adequate medical insurance can become literally a life-and-death difference; she may be unable to afford the preventive care she needs. Statistics prove this with macabre clarity. Low-income women, quite understandably, often must tolerate inadequate health care. One result is that those low-income women who develop breast cancer are diagnosed at later stages and die of cancer more frequently than other women. They suffer preventable death from breast cancer *two and a half times as often.*[1]

The same goes for cervical cancer, an even more scandalous gap because the Pap smear has been accepted worldwide for almost fifty years. Despite the tremendous drop in deaths from this almost wholly preventable disease, poor women still die of it twice as often as better-off women, almost entirely because of inadequate screening. As in breast cancer, low-income women are diagnosed at later, less treatable stages.

These women know about the Pap smear, we found in research in low-income communities in Forsyth County, North Carolina. But many do not understand that early detection can save their lives. Few realize that early diagnosis is a lifesaver, not a death warrant. And fewer still feel that they can do anything very effective to preserve their own health or believe that a physician is their partner.

Granted, of course, this attitude is far from the only obstacle that stands between poor women and routine gynecological care. Those without adequate medical coverage face many competing demands on their meager resources. They can't afford to visit the doctor for preventive care and usually seek medical attention only for specific, acute complaints. They generally get the preventive care they do receive only in connection with those visits. They have trouble traveling to clinics and have to endure long hours in waiting rooms.

But attitude is not a negligible obstacle. Time after time, these women said that nothing could be done about cancer, that treatments were costly, ineffective, and disfiguring—observations born of experience with relatives and friends diagnosed too late. And most bitterly and ironically of all, they believe that early diagnosis, far from saving lives, merely prolongs suffering.

That's why we need urgent political action to provide proper preventive care for all American women and save the lives of many of our mothers, daughters, sisters, and friends.


## THE LAST WORD

Political empowerment, personal empowerment—both will add to your feeling of strength and efficacy. Both can help you—and women everywhere—face the challenge of breast cancer. The first words in this book belonged to Abby, but the last are Irene's: "This breast cancer is something that all women face. It's something we all have to think about. But we have to remember something else, too: A woman can do anything she wants to do. She's got that power. But to do it, we've got to use our own intelligence; we've got to use our minds and our hearts and our spirits."

# Directory of Breast Centers

The following list of breast centers was provided by the National Consortium of Breast Centers, based on a two-year search conducted by Barbara Rabinowitz, R.N., L.C.S.W. Since the National Consortium of Breast Centers is not a certifying organization, the directory does not certify the included centers, but presents information each center has made available.

## EAST COAST

Breast Evaluation Unit
Comprehensive Cancer Center
University of Alabama at
  Birmingham
108 Basic Health Sciences
  Education Complex
University Station
Birmingham, AL 35294
205-934-3690

Betty Ford Comprehensive Breast
  Center
Columbia Hospital for Women
  Medical Center
2440 M Street, N.W.
Washington, DC 20037
202-293-6654

Georgetown Comprehensive Breast
  Center
Vincent T. Lombardi Cancer
  Center
Georgetown University Medical
  Center
3800 Reservoir Road, N.W.
Washington, DC 20007
202-342-2400

The Gertrude and Philip Strax
  Breast Cancer Detection Institute
Executive Court at Inverrary
4300 North University Drive
Suite E-200
Lauderhill, FL 33321
305-742-3500

The Breast Center of the Health
   Services Center
HCA Medical Center of Port St.
   Lucie
1700 S.E. Hillmore Drive
Port St. Lucie, FL 33452
305-335-8911

Breast Diagnostic Center
Humana Hospital of St. Petersburg
6499 38th Avenue North, Suite A-2
St. Petersburg, FL 33710
813-341-4890

Comprehensive Breast Center
Moffitt Cancer Center
12902 Magnolia Drive
Tampa, FL 33612
813-972-8480

The Breast Consultation Services
Johns Hopkins Oncology Center
600 North Wolfe Street
Baltimore, MD 21205
301-955-8893

Breast Evaluation Program
University of Maryland Cancer
   Center
22 South Greene Street
Baltimore, MD 21201
301-328-4490

Breast Health Center
New England Medical Center
750 Washington Street
Boston, MA 02111
617-956-5757

Breast Evaluation Center
Dana Farber Cancer Institute
44 Binney Street

Boston, MA 02115
617-732-3666

Breast Care Center
Beth Israel Hospital
330 Brookline Avenue
Brookline, MA 02215
617-735-2900

Faulkner Breast Centre
1153 Centre Street
Jamaica Plains, MA 02130

University of Massachusetts
Breast Clinic and Counseling Service
55 Lake Avenue North
Worcester, MA 01605
617-856-3112

Hitchcock Breast Center
Dartmouth-Hitchcock Medical Center
Hanover, NH 03756
603-646-8029

Comprehensive Breast Care Center
Cooper Hospital/University
   Medical Center
UMDNJ—Robert Wood Johnson
   Medical School
3 Cooper Plaza, Suite 411
Camden, NJ 06103
609-342-2474

The Comprehensive Breast Center
   of Robert Wood Johnson
   Medical School
UMDNJ—Robert Wood Johnson
   Medical School
1 Robert Wood Johnson Place, CN
   19
New Brunswick, NJ 08903
201-937-7868; 201-937-7867

Women's Breast Center
Mercer Medical Center
446 Bellevue Avenue
Trenton, NJ 08607
609-394-4045

Special Surveillance Breast Center
Memorial Sloan-Kettering Cancer
  Center
Memorial Hospital
1275 York Avenue
New York, NY 10021
212-794-5877

Center for the Early Detection of
  Breast Cancer
University of Rochester Cancer
  Center
Box 704
601 Elmwood Avenue
Rochester, NY 14642
716-275-7895

The Women's Center at St.
  Vincent Health Center
232 West 25th Street
Erie, PA 16544
814-452-5228

The Mammacare Program of the
  Hershey Medical Center
Pennsylvania State University,
Hershey Medical Center—Family
  Practice
500 University Drive
Hershey, PA 17033
717-534-8181

Breast Cancer Program at Albert
  Einstein Medical Center
Northern Division

York and Tabor Roads
Klein 101
Philadelphia, PA 19141
215-456-7383

Hospital of the University of
  Pennsylvania
Department of Radiology
3400 Spruce Street
Philadelphia, PA 19146
215-662-4033

Breast Evaluation Center of the
  Fox Chase Cancer Center
Central and Shelmire Avenues
Philadelphia, PA 19111
215-728-2646; 215-728-3001

University of South Carolina
  School of Medicine
Comprehensive Breast Center
2 Medical Park Road, Suite 402
Columbia, SC 29203
803-256-0308

The Women's Center
Cookeville General Hospital
142 West 5th Street
Cookeville, TN 38501
615-528-2541, ext. 328

Fort Sanders Comprehensive
  Breast Center
1901 Clinch Avenue
Knoxville, TN 37916
615-971-1624; 615-971-9625

Breast Clinic, Joint Cancer Clinic
Box 629, Medical College of
  Virginia
Richmond, VA 23298-0001
804-786-9992

# MIDWEST

Macneal Cancer Center
3340 South Oak Park Avenue
Berwyn, IL 60402
312-795-0300

Comprehensive Breast Center
1725 West Harrison Street, #802
Chicago, IL 60612
312-421-4800

University Breast Care Center
University of Health Sciences
Chicago Medical School
3333 Green Bay Road
North Chicago, IL 60064

St. Margaret's Diagnostic Breast
  Center
Wishard Memorial Hospital
Indiana University Medical Center
  Campus
1001 West 10th Street
Indianapolis, IN 46202
317-630-6266 (630-MAMO)

Allen Memorial Hospital
Breast Imaging Suite
1825 Logan Avenue
Waterloo, IA 50703
319-235-3715

McAuley Breast Care
Reichert Health Building
St. Joseph Mercy Hospital
Ann Arbor, MI 48106
313-572-5900

University of Michigan Breast Care
  Center
2nd Level Taubman Health Center

1500 Medical Center Drive
Ann Arbor, MI 48109
313-936-6000

Michigan Cancer Foundation
Breast Cancer Detection Center
4160 John Road, Suite 615
Detroit, MI 48201
313-833-7700

Samaritan Health Center Breast
  Imaging Services
5555 Conner
Detroit, MI 48213
313-579-4180

Oakland County Division of
  Health
Breast Cancer Detection/Education
  Center
27725 Greenfield Road
Southfield, MI 48076
313-424-7100

Share Breast Cancer Support
  Program
Barnes Hospital at Washington
  University Medical Center
4949 Barnes Hospital Plaza
St. Louis, MO 63110
314-362-5585

Breast Diagnostic Center
The Cleveland Clinic Foundation
9500 Euclid Avenue
Cleveland, OH 44106
216-444-6618

The Kettering Breast Evaluation
Centers
15 Southmoor Circle, N.E.
Kettering, OH 45429
513-299-0099

Oklahoma Breast Care Center
13509 North Meridian, Suite 6
Oklahoma City, OK 73120
405-755-2273

Center for Breast Diseases
#508 2325 South Harvard Street
Tulsa, OK 74114
918-742-1138

Susan G. Komen Breast Centers
3409 Worth Street, Suite 320
Dallas, TX 75246
214-820-2430

Gigi Griffiths Hill Breast Center
Presbyterian Hospital of Dallas
8200 Walnut Hill Lane
Dallas, TX 75231
214-891-2598

UTMB Cancer Center
Department of Surgery UTMB
Galveston, TX 77550
409-761-2490

Breast Diagnostic Center
Northeast Medical Center Hospital
18951 Memorial North
Humble, TX 77338
713-540-1720

Regional Breast Care Center
Odessa Women's and Children's
Hospital
520 East 6th, P.O. Box 4859
Odessa, TX 79760
915-334-8888

Center for Breast Screening
Hillcrest Baptist Medical Center
3115 Pine, Suite 606
Waco, TX 76708
713-756-8988

# WEST COAST

N.T. Enloe Hospital
Breast Screening Center
5th Avenue and the Esplanade
Chico, CA 95926
916-891-7445

Lybrand Mammography and
Education Center
Scripps Memorial Hospital
9888 Genesee Avenue
La Jolla, CA 92037
619-457-6224

Memorial Breast Evaluation Center
2865 Atlantic, Suite 204
Long Beach, CA 90806
213-595-3838

USC Cancer Center—Norris
Cancer Research Hospital
Breast Cancer Screening Clinic for
High Risk Women
1441 Eastlake
Los Angeles, CA 90033
213-224-6426

The Breast Health Center of
  Memorial Hospital Medical
  Center
1700 Coffee Road
Modesto, CA 95355
209-572-7207

UCI Breast Imaging Center
UCI Medical Center
101 City Drive
Orange, CA 92668
714-634-6175

Women's Health Center of Los
  Medanos Community Hospital
2260 Gladstone, Suite 6
Pittsburg, CA 94565
415-427-2025

Theodore Gildred Cancer Facility
University of California—San
  Diego Cancer Center
220 Dickinson Street
San Diego, CA 92103
619-543-3893

Breast Evaluation Center of San
  Francisco
25 Van Ness Avenue
San Francisco, CA 94102
415-621-5999

Breast Screening Center
University of California San
  Francisco
400 Parnassus Avenue, Room
  A-680

San Francisco, CA 94143
415-476-3282

Women's Care Breast Screening
  Center
480 Davis Court
San Francisco, CA 94611
415-781-6006

Breast Health Center of Children's
  Hospital of San Francisco
3700 California Street
San Francisco, CA 94118
415-387-8700, ext. 6366

Portland Adventist Mammography
  Services
Portland Adventist Medical Center
10123 S.E. Market
Portland, OR 97216
503-251-6132

Breast Evaluation Center
LDS Hospital
325 8th Avenue
Salt Lake City, UT 84103
801-321-1791

Group Health Corporation
5200 152nd N.E.
Redmond, WA 98052
206-882-5476

Breast Diagnostic Centers
411 Stronder Boulevard
Seattle, WA 98188
206-575-9123

# Recommended Reading

## Breast Health and Breast Cancer

*American Cancer Society.* Pamphlets on breast self-exam, dietary guidelines, and breast cancer. For materials and information contact your local American Cancer Society unit or state chartered division or call the national hotline: 1-800-ACS-2345. Address: American Cancer Society National Office, 15999 Clifton Road, NE, Atlanta, GA 30329. 404-320-3333.

Cooper, C. L. (1988). *Stress and breast cancer.* New York: John Wiley & Sons.

Kushner, R. (1984). *Alternatives—New developments in the war on breast cancer.* Cambridge, MA: Kensington Press.

Love, S. M., with Lindsey, K. (1990). *Dr. Susan Love's breast book.* Reading, MA: Addison-Wesley.

*NABCO News.* A quarterly newsletter published by the National Alliance of Breast Cancer Organizations addressing the latest in breast cancer research and treatments. For information on the publication and organization, write: NABCO, 1180 Avenue of the Americas, New York, NY 10036. 212-719-0154.

*National Cancer Institute.* Offers free information to the public on breast evaluation, breast biopsy, primary treatment, adjuvant therapy, follow-up care, breast reconstruction, recurrent disease, and advanced disease. For information or materials call the Cancer Information Service Hotline: 1-800-4-CANCER or write Office of Cancer Communications, National Cancer Institute, Building 31, Room 10 A 24, Bethesda, MD 20892.

National Cancer Institute, Office of Cancer Communications (1984). *The breast cancer digest: A guide to medical care, emotional support, educational programs, and resources* (2nd edition). Bethesda, MD: National Institutes of Health (NIH Publication #84-1691).

*National Consortium of Breast Centers.* Publishes *The Breast Center Bulletin* and *A Directory of Breast Centers.* Memberships available for individuals and organizations. Write: The National Consortium of Breast Centers, c/o The Comprehensive Breast Center, U.M.D.N.J.—R.W.J.M.S., 1 Robert Wood Johnson Place, CN 19, New Brunswick, NJ 08903-0019.

Seltzer, V. (1988). *Every woman's guide to breast cancer.* New York: Penguin Books.

Strax, P. (1989). *Make sure you do not have breast cancer.* New York: St. Martin's Press.

## DIET AND NUTRITION

American Health Foundation (1990). *Live well the low-fat/high-fiber way.* Valhalla, NY: American Health Foundation.

Committee on Diet and Health, National Research Council (1989). *Diet and health.* Washington, DC: National Academy Press.

Cooper, K. (1988). *Controlling cholesterol.* New York: Bantam Books.

Kaiser Permanente (1991). *Health counts. A fat and calorie guide.* New York: John Wiley & Sons.

Katahn, M. (1989). *The t-factor diet.* New York: Bantam Books.

Piscatella, J. C. (1991). *Controlling your fat tooth.* New York: Workman Publishing.

## EMOTIONAL SUPPORT/SELF-HELP

Burns, D. (1980). *Feeling good.* New York: William Morrow.

Burns, D. (1989). *The feeling good handbook.* New York: Penguin Group.

Beck, A. T., Rush, A. J., Shaw, B. F., & Emery, G. (1979). *Cognitive therapy of depression.* New York: Guilford Press.

Ellis, A., & Dryden, W. (1987). *The practice of rational-emotive therapy (RET).* New York: Springer Publishing Co.

Emery, G. (1988). *Getting un-depressed: How a woman can change her life through cognitive therapy*. New York: Simon & Schuster.

Walen, S. R., DiGiuseppe, R., & Wessler, R. L. (1980). *A practitioner's guide to rational-emotive therapy*. New York: Oxford University Press.

## EXERCISE

Kashiwa, A., & Rippe, J. (1987). *Fitness walking for women*. New York: Putnam Publishing Group.

Rippe, J. M., & Ward, A. (1989). *Dr. James M. Rippe's complete book of fitness walking*. New York: Prentice Hall Press.

*The Walking Magazine*. 9–11 Harcourt St., Boston, MA 02116. 1-800-678-0881 (U.S.) 303-666-7000 (Canada).

Yanker, G. D. (1983). *Rockport's complete book of exercise walking*. Chicago: Contemporary Books Inc.

## MOTHERS AND DAUGHTERS

Bassoff, E. (1988). *Mothers and daughters: Loving and letting go*. New York: New American Library.

Broner, E. M. (1975). *Her mothers*. Bloomington, IN: Indiana University Press.

Chernin, K. (1983). *In my mother's house*. New York: Harper & Row.

Friday, N. (1977, 1987). *My mother, my self: The daughter's search for identity*. New York: Dell.

Payne, K. (Ed.). (1983). *Between ourselves: Letters between mothers and daughters*. Boston: Houghton Mifflin.

## PSYCHOLOGY OF WOMEN

Baruch, G., & Brooks-Gunn, J. (Eds.). (1984). *Women in midlife*. New York: Plenum Press.

Chernin, K. (1986). *The hungry self: Women, eating, and identity*. New York: Harper & Row.

de Castillejo, I. C. (1973). *Knowing woman*. New York: Harper & Row.

Gilligan, C. (1982). *In a different voice: Psychological theory and women's development*. Cambridge, MA: Harvard University Press.

Harding, E. M. (1970). *The way of all women*. New York: Harper & Row.

Josselson, R. (1987). *Finding herself. Pathways to identity development in women*. San Francisco: Jossey-Bass.

McGrath, E., Keita, G. P., Strickland, B. R., & Russo, N. F. (1990). *Women and depression. Risk factors and treatment issues. Final report of the American Psychological Association's national task force on women and depression*. Washington, DC: American Psychological Association.

Walsh, M. R. (Ed.). (1987). *The psychology of women. Ongoing debates*. New Haven, CT: Yale University Press.

## Stress and Relaxation

Barnett, R. C., Biener, L., & Baruch, G. K. (Eds.). (1987). *Gender and stress*. New York: The Free Press.

Benson, H. (1976). *The relaxation response*. New York: Avon Books.

Benson, H. (1984). *Beyond the relaxation response*. New York: Times Books.

Borysenko, J. (1987). *Minding the body, mending the mind*. Reading, MA: Addison-Wesley.

Girdano, D. A., Everly, G. S., & Dusek, D.E. (1990). *Controlling stress and tension* (3rd edition). Englewood Cliffs, NJ: Prentice-Hall.

## Women's Health

Boston Women's Health Book Collective (1984). *The new our bodies, ourselves*. New York: Simon & Schuster.

Doress, P. B., & Siegal, D. L. (1987). *Ourselves, growing older*. New York: Simon & Schuster.

*National Women's Health Network*. Women's Health Information Clearinghouse with information packets available on forty-four topics in women's health. Memberships available that include *Net-*

*work News* published six times per year. Write to National Women's Health Network, 1325 G St., N.W. Washington, DC 20005. 202-347-1140.

Travis, C. B. (1988). *Women and health psychology. Biomedical issues.* Hillsdale, NJ: Lawrence Erlbaum Associates.

Travis, C. B. (1988). *Women and health psychology. Mental health issues.* Hillsdale, NJ: Lawrence Erlbaum Associates.

Wolfe, S. M. (1991). *Women's health alert.* Reading, MA: Addison-Wesley.

# References

## PREFACE

1. Royak-Schaler, R. (1992). Psychological processes in breast cancer: A review of selected research. *Journal of Psychosocial Oncology*, 9 (4).
2. Folch-Lyon, E. & J. F. (1981). Conducting focus group sessions. *Studies in Family Planning*, *12*, 443–449.
3. American Cancer Society (1991). *Cancer facts and figures—1991.* Atlanta, GA: American Cancer Society.

## CHAPTER 1

1. Adams-Greenly, M., & Moynihan, R. (1983). Helping the children of fatally ill parents. *American Journal of Orthopsychiatry*, *53*, 219–229.
2. Rosenfeld, A.; Caplan, G.; Yaroslavsky et al. (1983). Adaptation of children of parents suffering from cancer: A preliminary study of a new field for primary prevention research. *Journal of Primary Prevention*, *3*, 244–250.
3. Holland, J. C., & Rowland, J. H. (Eds.). (1989). *Handbook of psycho-oncology: Psychological care of the patient with cancer.* New York: Oxford University Press, pp. 588–595.
4. Brown, G. W., & Harris, T. (1978). *The social origins of depression: A study of psychiatric disorder in women.* London: Tavistock Publications.

CHAPTER 2

1. Lichtman, R. R.; Taylor, S. E.; Wood, J. V.; Bluming, A. S.; Dosik, G. M.; & Leibowitz, R. L. (1984). Relations with children after breast cancer: The mother-daughter relationship at risk. *Journal of Psychosocial Oncology, 2*, 1–19.

2. Bloom, J. R., & Psychological Aspects of Breast Cancer Study Group (1987). Psychological response to mastectomy: A prospective comparison study. *Cancer, 59*, 189–196.

3. Dean, C. (1987). Psychiatric morbidity following mastectomy: Preoperative predictors and type of illness. *Journal of Psychosomatic Research, 31*, 385–392.

4. Eisenberg, H. S., & Goldenberg, I. S. (1966). A measurement of quality of survival of breast cancer patients. In J. L. Hayward & R. D. Bulbrook (Eds.), *Clinical Evaluation of Breast Cancer* pp. (93–108). London: Academic Press.

5. Hughson, A. V. M.; Cooper, A. F.; McArdle, C. S.; & Smith, D. C. (1988). Psychosocial consequences of mastectomy: Levels of morbidity and associated factors. *Journal of Psychosomatic Research, 32*, 383–391.

6. Morris, T.; Greer, H. S.; & White, P. (1977). Psychological and social adjustment to mastectomy: A two-year follow-up study. *Cancer, 40*, 2381–2387.

7. Schottenfeld, F., & Robbins, G. F. (1970). Quality of survival among patients who have had radical mastectomy. *Cancer, 26*, 650–654.

8. Greer, S.; Morris, T.; & Pettingale, K. W. (1979). Psychological response to breast cancer: Effect on outcome. *Lancet, ii*, 785–787.

9. Pettingale, K. W.; Morris, T.; Greer, S.; & Haybittle, J. L. (1985). Mental attitudes to cancer: An additional prognostic factor. *Lancet, i*, 750.

10. Burgess, C.; Morris, T.; & Pettingale, K. W. (1988). Psychological response to cancer diagnosis—ll. Evidence for coping styles. *Journal of Psychosomatic Research, 32*, 263–272.

## CHAPTER 3

1. Williams, T. T. (1991). *Refuge*. New York: Viking Press.

## CHAPTER 4

1. Bishop, J. M. (1985). Oncogenes. In J. B. Wyngaarden & L. H. Smith (Eds.), *Cecil textbook of medicine, 17th ed.* (pp. 1066–1068). Philadelphia: Saunders.

2. National Cancer Institute, Office of Cancer Communications (1984). *The Breast cancer digest, 2nd ed.* Bethesda, MD: National Institutes of Health (NIH Publication No. 84–1691).

3. American Joint Committee (1982). *Manual for staging of cancer*. Philadelphia: Lippincott.

4. Journal of the National Cancer Institute (1988). Treatment alert issued for node-negative breast cancer. *Journal of the National Cancer Institute, 80,* 550–551.

5. McGuire, W. L. (1989). Adjuvant therapy of node-negative breast cancer. *New England Journal of Medicine, 320,* 525–527.

6. De Vita, V. T. (1989). Breast cancer therapy: Exercising all our options. *New England Journal of Medicine, 320,* 527–529.

7. American Cancer Society (1991). *Cancer facts and figures—1991.* Atlanta, GA: American Cancer Society.

8. Makuc, D. M.; Freid, V. M.; & Kleinman, J. C. (1989). National trends in the use of preventive health care by women. *American Journal of Public Health, 79,* 21–26.

9. Stanford, J. L., & Greenberg, R. S. (1989). Breast cancer incidence in young women by estrogen receptor status and race. *American Journal of Public Health, 79,* 71–73.

10. Strax, P. (1989). Control of breast cancer through mass screening: From research to action. *Cancer, 63,* 1881–1887.

11. Shapiro, S. (1989). Determining the efficacy of breast cancer screening. *Cancer, 63,* 1873–1880.

12. Love, R. R. (1989). Tamoxifen therapy in primary breast cancer: Biology, efficacy and side effects. *Journal of Clinical Oncology, 1,* 803–815.

13. Congressional Caucus for Women's Issues (June 28, 1991). Congress issues breast cancer challenge to medical researchers. *Update on Women and Family Issues in Congress, 11*, 10.

## CHAPTER 5

1. Henderson, I. C.; Harris, J. R.; Kinne, K. W.; Hellman, S. (1989). Cancer of the breast. In V. DeVita, S. Hellman, & S. Rosenberg (Eds.), *Cancer: Principles and practice of oncology, 3rd ed.* (pp. 1197–1214). Philadelphia: Lippincott.
2. Bassett, M. T., & Krieger, N. (1986). Social class and black-white differences in breast cancer survival. *American Journal of Public Health, 76*, 1400–1403.
3. McWhorter, W. P.; Schatzkin; A. G.; Horm, J. W.; & Brown, C. C. (1989). Contribution of socioeconomic status to black/white differences in cancer incidence. *Cancer, 63*, 982–987.
4. National Center for Health Statistics (1990). *Health, United States, 1989.* Hyattsville, MD: Public Health Service.
5. Leis, H. P. (1980). Risk factors for breast cancer: An update. *Breast, 6*, 21–27.
6. Adami, H. O.; Hansen, J.; Jung, B., & Rimsten, A. (1980). Familiality in breast cancer: A case-control study in a Swedish population. *British Journal of Cancer, 42*, 71–77.
7. Anderson, D. E. (1974). Genetic study of breast cancer: Identification of a high risk group. Cancer, *34*, 1090–1097.
8. Kelly, P. T. (1981). Refinements in breast cancer risk analysis. *Archives of Surgery, 116*, 364–365.
9. Brinton, L. A.; Williams, R. R.; & Hoover, R. N. (1979). Breast cancer risk factors among screening program participants. *Journal of the National Cancer Institute, 62*, 37–44.
10. Shimkin, M. E. (1979). *Contrary to nature.* Washington, DC: U.S. Department of Health, Education, and Welfare, p. 92.
11. Harlap, A. (1991). Oral contraceptives and breast cancer. *Journal of Reproductive Medicine, 36*, 374–395.
12. Olsson, H.; Moller, T. R.; & Ranstam, J. (1989). Early oral contraceptive use and breast cancer among premenopausal

women: Final report from a study in southern Sweden. *Journal of the National Cancer Institute, 81,* 1000–1004.

13. Schlesselman, J. J.; Staden, B. V.; Murray, P.; & Lai, S. (1988). Breast cancer in relation to early use of oral contraceptives. *Journal of the American Medical Association, 259,* 1828–1833.

14. Hulka, B. S. (1990). Hormone-replacement therapy and the risk of breast cancer. *CA—A Cancer Journal for Clinicians, 40,* 289–296.

15. Bergkvist, L.; Adami, H. O.; Persson, I.; Hoover, R.; & Schairer, C. (1989). The risk of breast cancer after estrogen and estrogen-progestin replacement. *New England Journal of Medicine, 321,* 293–297.

16. Gail, M. H.; Brinton, L. A.; Byar, D. P.; Corle, D. K.; Green, S. B.; Schairer, C.; & Mulvihill, J. J. (1989). Projecting individualized probabilities of developing breast cancer for white females who are being examined annually. *Journal of the National Cancer Institute, 81,* 1879–1886.

17. Armstrong, B., & Doll, R. (1975). Environmental factors and cancer incidence and mortality with special reference to dietary practices. *International Journal of Cancer, 15,* 617–631.

18. Wynder, R. L. (1980). Dietary factors related to breast cancer. *Cancer, 46,* 899–904.

19. Kelsey, J. L.; Fischer, D. B.; Holford, T. R.; et al. (1981). Exogenous estrogens and other factors in the epidemiology of breast cancer. *Journal of the National Cancer Institute, 67,* 327–333.

20. Ballard-Barbash, R. M.; Schatzkin, A.; Carter, C. L.; et al. (1990). Body fat distribution and breast cancer in the Framingham study. *Journal of the National Cancer Institute, 82,* 286–290.

21. Folsom, A. R.; Kaye, S. A.; Prineas, R. J.; et al. (1990). Increased incidence of carcinoma of the breast associated with abdominal adiposity in postmenopausal women. *American Journal of Epidemiology, 131,* 794–803.

22. Carroll, K. K. (1975). Experimental evidence of dietary factors and hormone-dependent cancers. *Cancer Research, 35,* 3374–3383.

23. Gorbach, S. L. (1984). Estrogens, breast cancer, and intestinal flora. *Reviews of Infectious Diseases, 6,* 585–590.

24. Frisch, R. E.; Wyshak, G.; Albright, N. L.; et al. (1985). Lower prevalence of breast cancer and cancers of the reproductive system among former college athletes compared to non-athletes. *British Journal of Cancer, 52,* 885–891.

25. Willett, W. C.; Stampfer, M. J.; Colditz, G. A.; & Rosner, B. A. (1987). Dietary fat and the risk of breast cancer. *New England Journal of Medicine, 316,* 22–28.

26. Willett, W. C.; Stampfer, M. J.; Colditz, G. A.; et al. (1987). Moderate alcohol consumption and the risk of breast cancer. *New England Journal of Medicine, 316,* 1174–1180.

27. Schatzkin, A.; Jones, D. Y.; Hoover, R. N.; Taylor, P. R.; et al. (1987). Alcohol consumption and breast cancer in the epidemiologic follow-up study of the first national health and nutrition examination survey. *New England Journal of Medicine, 316,* 1169–1173.

28. Love, S. M.; Gellman, R. S.; & Silen, W. (1982). Fibrocystic disease of the breast—a nondisease? *New England Journal of Medicine, 307,* 1010–1014.

29. Devitt, J. E. (1981). Clinical benign disorders of the breast and carcinoma of the breast. *Surgery, Gynecology & Obstetrics, 152,* 437–440.

30. Cole, P.; Elwood, J. M.; & Kaplan, S. D. (1978). Incidence rates and risk factors for benign breast disease. *American Journal of Epidemiology, 108,* 112–120.

31. Fisher, B., & Carbone, P. (1982). Breast cancer. In J. F. Holland & E. T. Frei, Jr. (Eds.), *Cancer medicine.* Philadelphia: Lea & Febiger.

32. Hutchinson, W. B.; Thomas, D. B.; Hamlin, W. B.; et al. (1980). Risk of breast cancer in women with benign breast disease. *Journal of the National Cancer Institute, 65,* 13–20.

33. Love, S. M., with Lindsey, K. (1990). *Dr. Susan Love's breast book.* Reading, MA: Addison-Wesley, pp. 81–87.

34. Page, D. L.; Vanderzwagg, R.; Rogers, L. W.; et al. (1978). Relationship between the component parts of fibrocystic disease complex and breast cancer. *Journal of the National Cancer Institute, 61,* 1055.

35. Stomper, P. C.; Gelman, R. S.; Meyer, J. E.; & Gross, G. S. (1990). New England mammography survey 1988: Public misconceptions of breast cancer incidence. *Breast Disease.*
36. American Cancer Society (1991). *Cancer facts and figures—1991.* Atlanta, GA: American Cancer Society.
37. Baker, L. H. (1982). Breast cancer detection demonstration project: Five-year summary report. *CA—A Cancer Journal for Clinicians, 32,* 194–225.
38. Kelly, P. T. (1987). Risk counseling for relatives of cancer patients: New information, new approaches. *Journal of Psychosocial Oncology, 5,* 65–79.
39. Gail, M. H.; Brinton, L. A.; Byar, D. P., et al. (1989). Projecting individualized probabilities of developing breast cancer for white females who are being examined annually. *Journal of the National Cancer Institute, 81,* 1184.

CHAPTER 6

1. American Cancer Society (1991). *Cancer facts and figures—1991.* Atlanta, GA: American Cancer Society.
2. Baines, C. J.; Miller, A. B.; & Bassett, A. A. (1989). Physical examination, its role as a single screening modality in the Canadian National Breast Screening Study. *Cancer, 63,* 1816–1822.
3. Shapiro, S. (1989). Determining the efficacy of breast cancer screening. *Cancer, 63,* 1873–1880.
4. Tabar, L.; Fagerberg, C. J. G.; Gad, A.; et al. (1985). Reduction in mortality from breast cancer after screening with mammography. *Lancet, 1,* 829–832.
5. Seidman, H.; Geib, S. K.; Silverbert, E.; et al. (1987). Survival experience in the Breast Cancer Detection Demonstration Project. *CA—A Cancer Journal for Clinicians, 37,* 258–290.
6. Jacobs Institute of Women's Health, National Cancer Institute, & Centers for Disease Control (1990). *Report of the Jacobs Institute workshop on increasing utilization of mammography screening by primary care providers.* Washington, DC: Jacobs Institute, p. 8.

7. Kuester, G. F., & Wolfe, S. M. (1991). *HRG report on screening mammography and ranking of eleven metro Washington area facilities*. Washington, DC: Public Citizen.

8. National Cancer Institute (1980). *National survey on breast cancer: A measure of progress in public understanding*. NIH Pub. No. 81-2306. Washington, DC: Government Printing Office.

9. Tannenbaum, A. (1942). Genesis and growth of tumors, III. Effects of high-fat diet. *Cancer Research, 2,* 468–475.

10. Hulka, B. S. (1989). Dietary fat and breast cancer: Case-control and cohort studies. *Preventive Medicine, 18,* 180–193.

11. MacMahon, B. (1979). Dietary hypotheses concerning the etiology of human breast cancer. *Nutrition and Cancer, 1,* 38–41.

12. Folsom, A. R.; Kaye, S. A.; Prineas, R. J.; et al. (1990). Increased incidence of carcinoma of the breast associated with abdominal adiposity in postmenopausal women. *American Journal of Epidemiology, 131,* 794–803.

13. Boyar, A. P.; Rose, D. P.; & Wynder, E. L. (1988). Recommendations for the prevention of chronic disease: The application for breast disease. *Amercian Journal of Clinical Nutrition, 48,* 896–900.

14. Willett, W. C.; Browne, M. L.; Bain, C.; et al. (1985). Relative weight and risk of breast cancer among premenopausal women. *American Journal of Epidemiology, 122,* 731–740.

15. Prentice, R. L.; Kakar, F.; Hursting, S.; et al. (1988). Aspects of the rationale of the Women's Health Trial. *Journal of the National Cancer Institute, 80,* 802–814.

16. Healy, B. (1991). Women's health, public welfare. *Journal of the American Medical Association, 266,* 566–568.

17. Boyd, N. F.; Cousins, M.; Beaton, M.; et al. (1988). Clinical trial of low-fat, high-carbohydrate diet in subjects with mammographic dysplasia: Report of early outcomes. *Journal of the National Cancer Institute, 80,* 1244–1253.

18. Boyd, N. F.; Shannon, P.; Kriukov, V.; et al. (1988). Effect of a low-fat high-carbohydrate diet on symptoms of cyclical mastopathy. *Lancet, 2* (8063), 128–132.

19. Folkins, C. H.; Lynch, S.; & Gardner, M. M. (1972). Psychological fitness as a function of physical fitness. *Archives of Physical Medicine and Rehabilitation, 53,* 503–508.
20. Morgan, W. P. (1981). Psychological benefits of physical activity. In F. Nagle & H. Montoye (Eds.), *Exercise, health and disease.* Springfield, IL: Thomas.
21. Doyne, E. J.; Chambless, D. L.; & Beutler, L. E. (1983). Aerobic exercise as a treatment for depression in women. *Behavior Therapy, 14,* 434–440.
22. Long, B. C., & Haney, C. J. (1988). Coping strategies for working women: Aerobic exercise and relaxation interventions. *Behavior Therapy, 19,* 75–83.
23. Greist, J. H.; Klein; M. H.; Eischens, R. R.; et al. (1979). Running as treatment for depression. *Comprehensive Psychiatry, 20,* 41–54.
24. Hiatt, R. A., & Bawol, R. D. (1984). Alcoholic beverage consumption and breast cancer incidence. *American Journal of Epidemiology, 120,* 676–683.
25. Willett, W. C.; Stampfer, M. J.; Colditz, G. A.; et al. (1987). Moderate alcohol consumption and the risk of breast cancer. *New England Journal of Medicine, 316,* 1174–1180.
26. Schatzkin, A.; Carter, C. L.; Green, S. B.; et al. (1989). Is alcohol consumption related to breast cancer? Results from the Framingham Heart Study. *Journal of the National Cancer Institute, 81,* 31–35.
27. Schatzkin, A.; Jones, D. Y.; Hoover, R. N.; et al. (1987). Alcohol consumption and breast cancer in the epidemiologic follow-up study of the first National Health and Nutrition Examination Survey. *New England Journal of Medicine, 316,* 1160–1173.
28. Harlap, S. (1991). Oral contraceptives and breast cancer. *Journal of Reproductive Medicine, 36,* 374–395.
29. McPherson, K.; Vessey, M. P.; Neil, A.; et al. (1987). Early oral contraceptive use and breast cancer: Results of another case-control study. *British Journal of Cancer, 56,* 653–660.
30. Kay, C. R., & Hannaford, P. C. (1988). Breast cancer and the pill—a further report from the Royal College of General Prac-

titioners' oral contraception study. *British Journal of Cancer, 58,* 675–680.

31. Olsson, H.; Moller, T. R.; & Ranstam, J. Early oral contraceptive use and breast cancer among premenopausal women: Final report from a study in southern Sweden. *Journal of the National Cancer Institute, 81,* 1000–1004.

32. Harris, N. V.; Weiss, N. S.; Francis, A. M.; et al. (1982). Breast cancer in relation to patterns of oral contraceptive use. *American Journal of Epidemiology, 116,* 643–651.

33. Schlesselman, J. J.; Stadel, B. V.; Murray, P.; & Lai, S. (1988). Breast cancer in relation to early use of oral contraceptives. *Journal of the American Medical Association, 259,* 1828–1833.

34. Stadel, B. V.; Lai, S.; Schlesselman, J. J.; et al. (1988). Oral contraceptives and premenopausal breast cancer in nulliparous women. *Contraception, 38,* 287–299.

35. Hulka, B. S. (1990). Hormone-replacement therapy and the risk of breast cancer. *CA—A Cancer Journal for Clinicians, 40,* 289–296.

36. Bergkvist, L.; Adami, H. O.; Persson, I.; et al. (1989). The risk of breast cancer after estrogen and estrogen-progestin replacement. *New England Journal of Medicine, 321,* 293–320.

37. Osborne, M. P., & Bayle, J. C. (1988). We would very rarely recommend prophylactic mastectomy. *Primary Care & Cancer, 8,* 25–31.

38. Humphrey, L. J. (1983). Subcutaneous mastectomy is not a prophylaxis against carcinoma of the breast: Opinion or knowledge? *American Journal of Surgery, 145,* 311–312.

CHAPTER 7

1. Taylor, Shelley E. (1986). *Health Psychology.* New York: Random House, pp. 240–263.

2. DiMatteo, M. R., & Friedman, H. S. (1982). *Social psychology and medicine.* Cambridge, MA: Oelgeschlager, Gunn, & Hain, pp. 81–115.

3. DiMatteo, M. R. (1979). A social-psychological analysis of physician-patient rapport: Toward a science of the art of medicine. In M. R. DiMatteo & Howard S. Friedman (Eds.) (1979).

Interpersonal relations in health care, *Journal of Social Issues, 35,* 12–33.

CHAPTER 9

1. Kash, K. M.; Holland, J. C.; Halper, M.; & Miller, D.G. (1991, April 10–12). Women at high genetic risk of breast cancer: Surveillance behavior and psychological distress. Paper presented at American Society of Preventive Oncology, Seattle, WA.
2. Royak-Schaler, R. (1990, August 13). Breast cancer's impact: Focus groups with high risk women. Paper presented at the American Psychological Association Convention, Boston, MA.
3. Folkman, S., & Lazarus, R. S. (1980). An analysis of coping in a middle-aged community sample. *Journal of Health and Social Behavior, 21,* 219–239.
4. Lazarus, R. S., & Folkman, S. (1984). *Stress, appraisal, and coping.* New York: Springer.
5. Szasz, S. (1991). *Living with it: Why you don't have to be healthy to be happy.* Buffalo, NY: Prometheus, p. 10.

CHAPTER 10

1. Thompson, S. C. (1981). Will it hurt less if I can control it? A complex answer to a simple question. *Psychological Bulletin, 90,* 89–101.
2. Bandura, A. (1977). Self-efficacy: Toward a unifying theory of behavior change. *Psychological Review, 84,* 191–215.
3. Bandura, A. (1982). Self-efficacy mechanism in human agency. *American Psychologist, 37,* 122–147.
4. DiClemente, C. D.; Prochaska, J. O.; & Gibertini, M. (1985). Self-efficacy and the stages of self-change of smoking. *Cognitive Therapy and Research, 9,* 181–200.
5. Kaplan, R. M.; Atkins, C. J.; & Reinsch, S. (1984). Specific efficacy expectations mediate exercise compliance in patients with COPD. *Health Psychologist, 3,* 223–242.
6. Marlatt, G. A., & Gordon, J. (1980). Determinants of relapse: Implications for the maintenance of behavior change. In P. Da-

vidson & S. Davidson (Eds.), *Behavioral* medicine: Changing health lifestyles (pp. 424–452). New York: Brunner/Mazel.

7. Gilchrist, L. D., & Schinke, S. P. (1983). Coping with contraception: Cognitive and behavioral methods with adolescents. *Cognitive Therapy and Research, 7*, 379–388.
8. Chambliss, C. A., & Murray, E. J. (1979). Efficacy attribution: Locus of control and weight loss. *Cognitive Therapy and Research, 3*, 349–353.
9. Strecher, V. J.; DeVellis, B. M.; Becker, M. H.; & Rosenstock, I. M. (1986). The role of self-efficacy in achieving health behavior change. *Health Education Quarterly, 13*, 73–91.
10. Doyne, E. J.; Chambless, D. L.; & Bentler, L. E. (1983). Aerobic exercise as a treatment for depression in women. Behavior Therapy, *14*, 434–440.

## CHAPTER 11

1. Ellis, A., & Dryden, W. (1987). *The practice of rational emotive therapy*. New York: Springer.
2. Ellis, A., & Harper, R. A. (1975). *A new guide to rational living*. North Hollywood, CA: Wilshire.
3. Burns, D. D. (1980). *Feeling good*. New York: Morrow, pp. 59–81.
4. Beck, A. T.; Rush, A. J.; Shaw, B. F.; & Emery, G. (1979). *Cognitive therapy of depression*. New York: Guilford, p. 403.
5. Benson, H. (1976). *The relaxation response*. New York: Aronson.
6. Borysenko, J. (1987). *Minding the body, mending the mind*. Reading, MA: Addison-Wesley.
7. Jacobson, E. (1978). *You must relax*. New York: McGraw-Hill.

## CHAPTER 12

1. American Cancer Society (1991). *Cancer facts and figures—1991*. Atlanta, GA: American Cancer Society.
2. Locker, A. P.; Caseldine, J.; Michell, A. K.; et al. (1989). Results from a seven-year programme of breast self-examination in 89,010 women. *British Journal of Cancer, 60*, 401–405.

3. National Cancer Institute, Office of Cancer Communications (1984). *Breast cancer digest, 2nd ed.* Bethesda, MD: National Institutes of Health (NIH Pub. No. 84–1691).

4. American Cancer Society (1987). *Special touch, a personal plan of action for breast health.* Brochure available from local chapters of the American Cancer Society or by calling 1-800-ACS-2345.

5. Cohen, L. A. (1987). Diet and cancer. *Scientific American, 257,* 42–48.

6. Reddy, B. S.; Hedges, A.; Laakso, K.; & Wynder, E. L. (1987). Metabolic epidemiology of large bowel cancer. Fecal bulk and constituents of high risk North Americans and low risk Finnish populations. *Cancer, 42,* 2832.

7. Rose, D. P.; Boyar, A. P.; Cohen, C.; & Strong, L. E. (1987). Effect of a low-fat diet on hormone levels in women with cystic breast disease. 1. Serum steroids and gonadotropins. *Journal of the National Cancer Institute, 78,* 623–626.

8. American Health Foundation (1990). *Live well the low-fat/high-fiber way. The American Health Foundation food plan.* New York: American Health Foundation.

9. American Cancer Society (1987). *Eating smart.* Booklet available from the American Cancer Society by calling 1-800-ACS-2345.

10. Blair, S. N.; Kohl, H. W.; Paffenbarger, R. S.; et al. (1989). Physical fitness and all-cause mortality. A prospective study of healthy men and women. *Journal of the American Medical Association, 262,* 2395–2401.

11. American College of Sports Medicine. (1978). *Sports Medicine Bulletin, 13,* 1–4.

12. Kashiwa, A., & Rippe, J. (1987). *Fitness walking for women.* New York: Putnam, pp. 45–63.

13. Blair, S. N.; Goodyear, N. N.; Gibbons, L. W.; & Cooper, K. H. (1984). Physical fitness and incidence of hypertension in healthy normotensive men and women. *Journal of the American Medical Association, 252,* 487–490.

14. Pocock, N. A.; Eisman, J. A.; Yeates, M. G.; et al. (1986). Physical fitness is a major determinant of femoral neck and lumbar

spine bone mineral density. *Journal of Clinical Investigation, 78,* 618–621.

15. McArdle, W. D.; Katch, F. I.; & Katch, V. L. (1981). *Exercise physiology.* Philadelphia: Lea & Febiger.

16. Wilkes, M. M.; Watkins, W. B.; Stewart, R. D.; & Yen, S. S. C. (1980). Localization and quantitation of beta-endorphin in human brain and pituitary. *Neuroendocrinology, 30,* 113–121.

17. Prior, J. C.; Vigna, Y.; Sciarretta, D.; et al. (1987). Conditioning exercise decreases premenstrual symptoms: A prospective, controlled 6-month trial. *Fertility and Sterility, 47,* 402–408.

18. Cohen, L. A. (1988). Reducing the risk of breast cancer. *Nutrition Action Healthletter, 15,* 4–6. Publication of the Center for Science in the Public Interest, Washington, DC.

AFTERWORD: REALISTIC RESPONSIBILITY

1. McWhorter, W. P.; Schatzkin, A. G.; Horm, J. W.; & Brown, C. C. (1989). Contribution of socioeconomic status to black/white differences in cancer incidence. *Cancer, 63,* 982–987.

# Index